Unlocking True Relief

Why Fascial Counterstrain Works When Physical Therapy, Massage, & Chiropractic Medicine Have Failed

Keryn Gold, PhD, MBA

Second Edition · Lead With Gold, LLC

Copyrights

Author: Keryn Gold, PhD, MBA
Publisher: Lead With Gold, LLC

Legal Disclaimer

This publication is intended to provide accurate and authoritative information regarding the subject matter covered. However, it is sold with the understanding that neither the author nor the publisher is engaged in rendering medical, legal, financial, insurance, accounting, or other professional services.

This book is not medical advice. It provides general information about chronic pain, manual therapy, and self-directed health practices. It is not a diagnosis, it is not a treatment recommendation for any individual, and reading it does not create a clinician relationship of any kind.

While every effort has been made to ensure the accuracy and completeness of the information in this book, the author and publisher make no guarantees, express or implied, regarding its applicability, reliability, or effectiveness for your individual circumstances. The approaches described may not be suitable for all individuals. Readers should seek professional guidance where appropriate.

Nothing in this book is a promise of relief. Outcomes depend on condition, history, practitioner, timing, and dozens of variables no author controls.

Neither the publisher nor the author shall be held liable for any direct, indirect, incidental, consequential, or other damages arising from the use of or reliance on this book's content, including but not limited to health outcomes, financial loss, legal disputes, or personal and professional consequences.

Seek Care First

Talk to a licensed clinician who knows your case before starting, stopping, or changing anything, including any medication, exercise program, or course of treatment.

Some symptoms need urgent medical evaluation rather than a book. These include new or progressive weakness, numbness in the groin or saddle area, any change in bladder or bowel control, fever with back pain, unexplained weight loss, a personal history of cancer, pain following significant trauma, chest pain, shortness of breath, or a new severe headache.

If any of those apply, contact a physician today.

Responsibility and Risk

By reading this book, you acknowledge that:

- You are solely responsible for your decisions, actions, and outcomes.
- The author and publisher do not accept liability for any health, financial, or legal results based on the material provided.
- The therapies, practices, and programs described are not endorsed, warranted, or supervised by the author or publisher, and no representation is made about any individual practitioner, clinic, organization, or company named in these pages.
- Any case studies, examples, and statistics are either drawn from publicly available data or represent composite stories drawn from real experience, with details changed to protect confidentiality.

Legal Notice

By continuing to read, you agree to these terms and assume full responsibility for how you apply the information presented.

About the Evidence in This Book

Every figure has a source at the back. Where a figure comes from an organization that sells the thing being measured, that is stated in the sentence rather than buried in a footnote. This happens more than once in these pages, including for Fascial Counterstrain itself.

Two kinds of examples appear here, and they should be distinguishable on sight. Published research is cited by author, journal, year, and sample size, with its limitations stated alongside it. Illustrative examples are composites built from patterns commonly described in this work, with details invented, and each one says so where it appears.

Descriptions of training programs, course sequences, directories, and prices reflect publicly available information at the time of writing and change without notice. Verify current details with the organization directly.

Disclosure

The author runs Save with Benefits, which helps employers make care affordable for their people. Chapter 8 describes a remote musculoskeletal care program that employers can offer, and that business can arrange access to such a program at negotiated rates. That is a direct financial interest, it is marked where it appears, and the evidence for that program is presented on the same terms as every other program in this book, including the parts that do not flatter it.

No company, clinic, or training organization named in this book paid for placement, reviewed the text, or knew it was being written.

No public figure named in this book reviewed it, endorsed it, or was paid in connection with it.

Paperback ISBN: 978-1-967456-19-2
Hardcover ISBN: 978-1-967456-20-8
eBook ISBN: 978-1-967456-18-5

First Edition, 2025
Second Edition, revised and expanded, 2026

LeadWithGold.com

Contents

Introduction

How long have you been living with pain?

If the answer is measured in years, I'm sorry. I know what that does to a person, because it did it to me. Not the pain itself so much as everything that grows around it. The plans that quietly stop getting made. The things that used to be an easy yes. The slow, private arithmetic of what a weekend is going to cost on Monday.

I lived with knee pain for 20 years. I'd had it since I was a teenager, and somewhere along the way I stopped calling it a problem and started calling it my knee. That's what can happen. It stops being something to solve and becomes part of the furniture.

Then a friend 20 years my senior told me about Fascial Counterstrain.

I'm a scientist. My PhD is in biomedical sciences, and my instinct when someone touts a technique I've never heard of is to go and read what's actually been published. So I was skeptical, the way I imagine anyone would be who's been dealing with pain for decades and thought they'd already tried everything.

I read the literature first. I found it thinner than the enthusiasm around it, and more interesting than I expected. Then I went anyway, because the downside was one appointment.

The pain resolved. Not managed, not quieter on good days. Gone, after the first appointment. Within weeks I was playing sports again, something I'd quietly stopped doing years before. I went back later for longstanding back pain and that resolved too.

I want to be careful here, because this is the moment where most books start selling you something.

I'm one person. One person is not evidence. I don't know whether your pain will respond the way mine did, or whether I happened to find an unusually good practitioner. The controlled research on this technique is small and early, and Chapter 4 says exactly how small, names every study, and flags who funded them.

What I can tell you is why almost nobody has heard of this, and it isn't anyone's failure. Not yours, not your doctor's. The systems that surface treatment options can only surface what's already inside them, and a technique taught in multiday post-graduate courses to a relatively small pool of clinicians has nowhere to appear in a short appointment. That's a structural gap, not a verdict on anybody.

That said, awareness is growing. As I write this, the Counterstrain Academy clinic finder lists practitioners in 41 states and the District of Columbia, and in 8 countries across 4 continents. There's a reasonable chance somebody trained in this works closer to you than you'd guess.

So this book does two things. It explains what this technique is and what the evidence does and doesn't support, and it gives you everything else that holds up under a clinical trial, including several things you can start tonight for free.

You get to decide for yourself. That's the whole point of writing it down.

How to read this

This book is built so you can skip straight to whatever you actually need.

Every chapter stands alone. Each opens with a 60-second version that tells you the decision it helps you make, the 4 questions it answers, and what you walk away with. Each closes with a playbook you can copy, send to someone, or run this week.

The book covers one therapy in depth, then widens. Fascial Counterstrain is the technique most people in chronic pain have never had visibility or access to, so it gets the first seven chapters. The last three cover what else holds up under a clinical trial, including things you can do at home for free.

Start wherever your problem is

↳ Tried everything, nothing held? Chapter 1.

↳ Want to understand the mechanism before you spend a dollar? Chapters 2 and 3.

↳ Want to see the actual studies and the holes in them? Chapter 4.

↳ Wondering whether your specific condition is even in scope? Chapter 5.

↳ Ready to book, and want to not waste the first session? Chapter 6.

↳ Worried about cost and how many visits this becomes? Chapter 7.

↳ Want something you can start tonight, for free? Chapters 8 and 9.

↳ A clinician deciding whether to train in this? Chapter 10.

Four ways to read it, by how you work

Few people read a book the way the author imagined. Pick the entry that matches how you operate.

Want the decision and the number, now. Read the 60-second block at the top of each chapter and the playbook at the bottom. Skip everything in between. That's about 20 minutes for the whole book.

Want the story and the people. Read Chapter 1, then Chapter 5, then the Conclusion. They carry the arc, and the rest supports them.

Want to be sure nothing blows up in your face. Start with Chapter 4, Chapter 7, and the safety sections in Chapters 5 and 9. Those are the risk chapters: what the evidence actually supports, what it costs, and which popular advice isn't as safe as it sounds.

Want the mechanism and the sources. Read Chapter 2, Chapter 3, and the references at the back first, then decide whether to trust the rest. That's the order I'd use, and it's the order I used.

Two notes on numbers

Every figure in this book has a source at the back. Where a figure comes from a company or an institute that sells the thing being measured, I say so in the sentence, not in a footnote.

Some of the best-known numbers in pain care are weaker than they sound. I'd rather hand you a number with its limits attached than a confident one you can't check.

One note on the subtitle

The subtitle says treatment has failed. Treatments fail. People don't.

A course of physical therapy that didn't hold was aimed at a real problem by someone doing the job properly, and the fact that it helped and then stopped tells you something useful about where to look next.

Specialists go deep. Going deep is exactly what makes them good at the job.

About the rest of the subtitle. "Science-backed" means published research exists, and Chapter 4 lays out all of it, holes included. "Safe" means the published studies report no serious adverse events, which isn't the same as risk-free for every person, and it's why the red flags in Chapter 5 come first. "Celebrities" refers to public testimonials like the one discussed in Chapter 4. None of those people reviewed or endorsed this book.

If the root cause of your pain were resolved, what would you do first?

PART ONE

What Is Actually Happening

CHAPTER 1

Why Has Everything I've Tried Been a Temporary Solution at Best?

Because almost everything on offer is aimed at the symptom, and the symptom isn't the cause. Treat where it hurts and it comes back. Find what's actually driving it, and it may not.

Why has everything you've tried been a temporary solution at best?

That question has a real answer, and it's a more hopeful one than most people expect. Relief that runs out isn't a sign that nothing works on you. It means something got to a real problem and stopped short of the thing producing it.

Which is good news, because a cause that hasn't turned up yet is a very different situation from a body that can't be helped.

> ## Start Here: The 60-Second Version
>
> **The decision this chapter helps you make.**
> Whether to keep managing this, or go looking for what's actually causing it.
>
> **The questions it answers.**

> ↳ Why has everything I've tried only worked for a while?
>
> ↳ Is this just aging, and is "wear and tear" even a real explanation?
>
> ↳ Why do imaging results so often not match the pain?
>
> ↳ What would a different model of chronic pain even look like?
>
> **Why it matters.** In 2023, about 1 in 4 U.S. adults (24.3%) lived with chronic pain, and about 1 in 12 (8.5%) had pain that often limited life or work, according to the CDC's National Center for Health Statistics. In chronic back pain specifically, about 85% of cases are classified as primary, meaning no clear peripheral cause is identified on examination or imaging. That isn't a small exception. That's most people.
>
> **What you walk away with.** A working explanation for why it keeps coming back, and the one question that tells you whether a practitioner is aiming at the cause or at the symptom.

Why it keeps coming back

A common pattern in long-term pain goes like this.

Something helps. A massage, a dry needling session, an adjustment, a new exercise. The relief is real, and it lasts a few hours or a few days.

Then it comes back, usually to exactly the same spot, sometimes worse.

It's easy to read that as "nothing works for me," or to wonder whether you didn't do enough of the exercises. A kinder and more accurate reading is that the intervention reached a real problem, just not the one producing it. Muscle tension that reappears in the same place on the same schedule is often being held there by something that never got addressed.

Why "wear and tear" is a weaker explanation than it sounds

The most common thing people are told is that this is age.

It's worth knowing how poorly imaging findings track with pain. In a systematic review of imaging in people with **no back pain at all**, published in the American Journal of Neuroradiology in 2015, disc degeneration appeared in 37% of asymptomatic 20-year-olds and 96% of asymptomatic 80-year-olds. Disc bulges appeared in 30% of asymptomatic 20-year-olds and 84% of asymptomatic 80-year-olds.

The overwhelming majority of pain-free 80-year-olds have degenerative changes on film.

Those findings are common features of a lived-in body, not reliable explanations for a specific pain. Which means a scan that shows degeneration hasn't necessarily found your problem. It has found something almost everyone your age has.

Is it too late at 70, or 80?

In the review above, 96% of pain-free 80-year-olds showed disc degeneration on imaging. So a scan full of "age-related changes" says less about what's still possible than it seems to.

Age can slow healing. It doesn't switch it off. Practitioners report resolving pain in people in their 70s and 80s that's been there for decades. That's clinical report, not a trial, and it's still worth knowing if anyone has told you it's too late.

What imaging is very good at, and what it isn't

None of this makes imaging useless. It's excellent at what it was built for: fractures, tumors, infection, nerve root compression severe enough to warrant surgery, structural instability. If a clinician orders a scan, there's a reason, and this book isn't an argument against it.

The limit is narrower and more specific. Imaging is poor at telling you which of several common findings is producing today's pain, because it can't see tissue irritation in the connective tissue that surrounds and separates everything else.

My scan is normal, so why does it still hurt?

So you end up in a strange middle zone.

The scan is unremarkable, or it shows the same changes as everyone else your age. Bloodwork is fine. Nobody can name a cause, so the plan becomes management: medication, periodic sessions, activity modification, and a slow narrowing of what feels possible.

The word that shows up in this zone is "idiopathic," which is medicine being honest that it doesn't have the mechanism. It isn't a dismissal, and the pain is just as real. It's an accurate description of a gap.

Chapter 2 is about the tissue that sits in that gap.

The one question worth asking before any treatment

Before you book anything, including Counterstrain, ask the practitioner this:

"What tissue do you think is generating this, and how will we know within one or two sessions whether you were right?"

A good answer names a structure and a timeline. A weak answer describes a package of visits.

This question isn't about catching anyone out. It's about whether the plan has a testable hypothesis in it, because a plan with a hypothesis can be wrong fast and cheap, and a plan without one can absorb a year.

Your Playbook

Copy this section and send it. It stands on its own, with no context from the rest of the book.

1. Write down every injury and surgery you've had, including the ones you think are irrelevant

Owner: You · Time: 15 min

2. Note how long relief lasted after each past treatment, in hours or days

Owner: You · Time: 10 min

3. Rule out red flags with a physician: new weakness, saddle numbness, bladder or bowel changes, unexplained weight loss, fever, cancer history

Owner: Your physician · Time: 1 visit

4. Ask any prospective practitioner the tissue-and-timeline question above

Owner: You · Time: 2 min

5. Read Chapter 3 before your first appointment so you know what a session should look like

Owner: You · Time: 12 min

The 3 rules that make it work.

1. **How long the relief lasts tells you the most.** A few hours means it treated the symptom. A few weeks usually means it got closer to the cause.
2. **An old injury can matter more than it seems.** The ankle you sprained at 17 belongs on the list.

3. **Rule out the dangerous things first.** Everything in this book assumes a physician has already cleared the serious causes.

How you'll know it's working in 30 days. You can state, in one sentence, what tissue a practitioner thinks is driving your pain. If nobody can answer that, you've learned something valuable about where to spend your next appointment.

Which old injury on your list surprised you most once you wrote it down?

CHAPTER 2

What Is Fascia, and Why Would It Be the Thing Generating Pain?

Fascia is the continuous connective tissue that wraps and separates every muscle, nerve, vessel, and organ. It's densely innervated, it drains through the lymphatic system, and when drainage stalls, inflammatory chemistry sits in it.

If a tissue ran through your entire body and could hurt, would you expect the pain to stay put?

Start Here: The 60-Second Version

The decision this chapter helps you make.
Whether the fascial model explains your pattern well enough to be worth testing.

The questions it answers.

- ↳ What is fascia, in plain language?
- ↳ Why would connective tissue generate pain rather than just hold things together?
- ↳ What does "interstitium" mean and why did it make the news?

> ↳ Why does pressing one spot reproduce pain somewhere else?
>
> **Why it matters.** Fascia contains sensory nerve endings in high density, which is why it can act as a pain generator rather than passive packing material. In 2018, a team publishing in Scientific Reports described the interstitium, the fluid-filled space within and between connective tissue layers, as a continuous, fluid-carrying network that standard tissue-slide preparation had been collapsing and therefore hiding for decades.
>
> **What you walk away with.** An explanation simple enough to remember, and enough of the vocabulary to tell whether a practitioner is describing something real.

The simple version

Imagine a bodysuit made of webbing. Now imagine it doesn't stop at your skin. It continues inward, wrapping each muscle, then each bundle inside that muscle, then each fiber. It sleeves your nerves. It forms the outer coat of your arteries. It suspends and separates your organs.

That's fascia. If you removed every bone and organ and kept only the fascia, you would still have a recognizable human shape.

Two properties make it relevant to pain.

It's continuous. There's no clean boundary where your calf's fascia stops and your hamstring's begins. Tension is transmitted, not contained.

It's innervated. Fascia carries free nerve endings and mechanoreceptors in high density, including nociceptors, the endings that signal potential tissue threat. A structure with nociceptors in it can generate pain. That's what nociceptors do.

The interstitium, and why it matters here

In March 2018, Benias and colleagues published a paper in Scientific Reports describing the interstitium in human tissue as a network of fluid-filled spaces supported by collagen bundles, present throughout the body and draining into the lymphatic system.

The finding wasn't that a new organ had appeared. It was that standard histology slides, which are dehydrated during preparation, had been collapsing these fluid spaces flat. Once researchers looked at living tissue with confocal laser endomicroscopy, the spaces were visibly open and fluid was moving through them.

This matters for pain for one reason. If fluid moves through connective tissue, then fluid can also fail to move through connective tissue.

Where the Counterstrain model picks up

In 2021, Tuckey and colleagues published a mechanism paper in Frontiers in Pain Research proposing that impaired lymphatic drainage and stagnant inflammatory fluid in the interstitium could sustain chronic pain.

The proposed chain runs like this.

1. Tissue injury or an immune response releases inflammatory mediators into the interstitial space.
2. Some of those mediators, including interleukin-1 beta, interleukin-6, and tumor necrosis factor alpha, also impair the pumping of lymphatic vessels. Another, TGF-beta 1, encourages connective tissue cells to contract.
3. Contracted tissue and sluggish lymphatics slow the drainage of the same inflammatory mediators that caused the slowdown.
4. The chemistry stays put. Local nociceptors stay chemically activated. The nervous system keeps receiving a threat signal from a place where the original injury healed years ago.

Picture a garden hose with a kink in it. The water's still there. It just can't get through, and pressure builds behind the bend. The drainage model proposes something similar in connective tissue: fluid that should move on stalls, and the chemistry that irritates nerves stays put.

It's worth being precise about what that paper is. It's a theoretical mechanism review, not a clinical trial. It proposes an explanation and assembles supporting physiology from other research. It doesn't, by itself, demonstrate that treating fascia relieves pain. The lead author developed Fascial Counterstrain and owns a clinic that provides it, which is worth weighing alongside the argument.

I include it because a treatment with a stated, falsifiable mechanism is a better bet than one without. Not because a mechanism paper settles anything.

Why pressing here reproduces pain there

This is the part that tends to convince people, and it has a boring anatomical explanation.

Nerves from deep structures and nerves from skin converge on the same segments of the spinal cord. When a deep structure is chemically irritated, the brain can misattribute the signal to the skin region that shares that spinal segment. That's referred pain, and it's the same mechanism that puts heart attack pain in the left arm.

The practical consequence is that the surface spot that hurts and the deep tissue generating the signal can be far apart, and reliably so. The referral patterns are mapped, which is why a trained practitioner presses your abdomen when you came in about your neck.

What the model doesn't claim

Being fair to the model means being clear about its edges.

↳ It doesn't claim fascia explains all pain. Fractures, infection, tumors, inflammatory arthritis, and nerve root compression are real, distinct, and need real, distinct treatment.

↳ It doesn't claim that a session "breaks up adhesions." That older explanation, still repeated widely, isn't what the current model describes and isn't mechanically plausible with the forces involved.

↳ It doesn't claim results are permanent. A resolved restriction can be re-established by a new injury or a new inflammatory event.

Your Playbook

Copy this section and send it. It stands on its own, with no context from the rest of the book.

> **1.** Map your pain: where it starts, where it travels, what makes it move
>
> *Owner: You · Time: 10 min*

> **2.** List surgeries and abdominal or pelvic procedures, including C-sections and appendectomies
>
> *Owner: You · Time: 5 min*

> **3.** Note any non-musculoskeletal symptoms alongside the pain: bloating, dizziness on standing, swelling, headaches
>
> *Owner: You · Time: 5 min*

> **4.** Ask a prospective practitioner to explain the mechanism in their own words
>
> *Owner: You · Time: 5 min*

> **5.** Compare their answer to this chapter. Drainage and inflammation is the current model. "Breaking up adhesions" is the retired one
>
> *Owner: You · Time: 2 min*

The 3 rules that make it work.

1. **The fascia runs through everything, and that's the whole point.** If a practitioner only examines the spot that hurts, they aren't working from this model.
2. **Referred pain is normal, not mysterious.** Convergence at the spinal cord explains it.
3. **An explanation isn't the same thing as evidence.** Chapter 4 is where the evidence gets weighed.

How you'll know it's working in 30 days. You can explain to a skeptical friend, in two sentences, what this model proposes and what it doesn't.

Which of your symptoms have you been treating as separate problems, and what would change if they shared one cause?

CHAPTER 3

What Is Counterstrain, and What Actually Happens in a Session?

A practitioner finds tender points that map to specific deep structures, shortens the tissue around each one for roughly 30 to 90 seconds, and rechecks. There's no force, no thrust, and no pain during the technique.

What would change if you knew, before you booked, exactly what the hour would look like?

> ## Start Here: The 60-Second Version
>
> **The decision this chapter helps you make.**
> Whether this is a treatment you would be comfortable trying.
>
> **The questions it answers.**
>
> ↳ Where did this technique come from?
>
> ↳ What's the difference between Strain-Counterstrain and Fascial Counterstrain?
>
> ↳ What physically happens to me during an appointment?
>
> ↳ How will I know within one session whether anything changed?

Why it matters. In the one randomized study of Fascial Counterstrain published to date, three sessions of 90 minutes were delivered over an average of 19.5 days, and no adverse events were reported in either the treatment or the control group. Whatever else is uncertain, the risk profile of a no-force technique is low, and that changes the calculus of trying it.

What you walk away with. A clear picture of the hour, and one objective test you can run on yourself.

Where it came from

In the 1950s, an osteopathic physician named Lawrence Jones had a patient with severe low back pain who hadn't responded to treatment. He positioned the man for comfort while he considered what to do next, left him there, and returned to find the pain substantially reduced.

That accident became a method. Jones spent years mapping tender points and the positions that quieted them, and published Strain and Counterstrain. He and Randall Kusunose founded the Jones Institute in 1988 to teach it.

The mechanism Jones proposed, involving muscle spindles, has since been argued against within the field itself. That's normal scientific progress and not a mark against the technique. What survived was the clinical observation: a specific position, held briefly, reliably quiets a specific tender point.

Strain-Counterstrain versus Fascial Counterstrain

These are two different things and the distinction matters when you read research, because studies of one don't automatically support the other.

Strain-Counterstrain (SCS) is the original osteopathic method. Roughly 200 techniques, focused on the musculoskeletal system, taught across two main courses. This is the version with the most published trial data.

Fascial Counterstrain (FCS) is the later expansion, developed by Brian Tuckey, a physical therapist and one of a small number of people certified directly by Jones. FCS adds over 900 techniques across six anatomical systems: musculoskeletal, lymphatic-venous, arterial, visceral, and nervous system, plus a central sensitization series. The treatment positions are described as fascial glides applied to deep structures rather than the classic Jones positions of comfort.

The practical difference for you: FCS practitioners can address vascular, visceral, and nervous system tissue that a classic SCS practitioner isn't trained to treat. That's why the reported condition list is so much wider, and also why a curious reader should hold the wider claims to a higher standard.

What an appointment actually looks like

You stay fully clothed. Loose or stretchy clothing. Athletic wear is ideal.

The history is long. Expect 20 to 40 minutes on your first visit, covering injuries you think are irrelevant, every surgery, car accidents, falls, and illnesses. A practitioner working from this model needs the whole timeline, because whatever is causing this may be decades old and nowhere near where it hurts.

The scan comes next. The practitioner palpates a sequence of surface points, usually across your whole body, not just the painful region. Tender points in this model are described as small, roughly 1 cm areas of tissue that feel tense, slightly swollen, and sharply tender compared to the tissue around them.

Some of them tend to surprise people. That's expected, and it's the referred-pain convergence from Chapter 2, not magic.

Then treatment. For each point, the practitioner moves you into a position that slackens the tissue around it, or applies a light manual glide to a deeper structure. You hold. The published protocol in the post-traumatic stress disorder (PTSD) study held each release 30 to 45 seconds. In general practice, 30 to 90 seconds is the common range.

It shouldn't hurt. If a technique is painful, say so. The whole premise of this method is that the tissue lets go when it isn't being fought.

It's closer to untangling a knotted shoelace than pulling it tight. Yank the ends and the knot locks. Ease them toward each other and there's room for it to loosen.

Then the recheck. The practitioner presses the same point again. Either it has changed or it hasn't. That immediate recheck is useful feedback, with one caveat: tender points can soften with almost any gentle contact, so a point that changes on the table isn't proof on its own. The movement test below, run over several days, tells you more.

A common first reaction is some version of "wait, that's it?" The technique is that light, and that's the point.

Then they move on. A session typically works through a sequence of points, and a first session commonly runs 60 to 90 minutes.

What it feels like afterward

Most people report feeling relaxed to the point of drowsiness. Some report a mild soreness, like the day after unfamiliar exercise, lasting a day or so. Some feel a change in a symptom they didn't mention.

Is it normal to feel sore, or even worse, afterward? Often, and briefly. A 2010 systematic review of hands-on therapies found mild to moderate reactions after about 41% of treatments in cohort studies and 22% in randomized trials, at rates similar to exercise and placebo. Serious events were rare, around 0.13%. That review wasn't specific to Counterstrain, and no Counterstrain-specific safety study exists yet. The Fascial Counterstrain trial in Chapter 4 reported no adverse events in either group.

When is it worth a call? Anything on the red-flag list in Chapter 5, new numbness or weakness, or pain that's clearly worse and still climbing after about 3 days. That 3-day line is a common clinical rule of thumb, not a research finding.

What about emotions? Counterstrain's own website notes that some people experience strong memories during or after treatment aimed at stress and trauma. For anyone with a trauma history, telling the practitioner beforehand, and keeping a mental health clinician in the loop, can make the experience feel a lot safer.

Practitioners commonly suggest water, an easy day, and paying attention over the next 48 hours.

Practitioners working this way rarely hand out an exercise sheet. The approach is built on doing less, not more.

The one objective test to run on yourself

Testimonials are unreliable, and memory of yesterday's pain is less reliable than it feels. So measure something.

Pick one movement you can repeat exactly: how far you can turn your head before it catches, how far down your shin you can reach, how long you can stand before the ache starts.

Record it the morning of your appointment. Record it the next morning. Record it a week later.

That's a crude measurement, and it's still far better than asking yourself whether you feel better.

How is it different from massage, chiropractic, or dry needling?

Each of these is aimed at something real, and specialists in each go deep. The difference is where they aim.

Fascial Counterstrain

↳ Force: None; positioning and light glides

↳ Painful during? Shouldn't be

↳ Aims at: Tender points linked to deeper tissue, often away from the pain

Massage

↳ Force: Light to deep pressure

↳ Painful during? Can be, with deep work

↳ Aims at: Muscle near the pain

Myofascial release

↳ Force: Sustained pressure and stretch

↳ Painful during? Can be

↳ Aims at: Fascia and muscle near the pain

Craniosacral therapy

↳ Force: Very light touch

↳ Painful during? Shouldn't be

↳ Aims at: Mostly the head, spine, and pelvis

Muscle energy technique

↳ Force: Your own gentle contraction against the practitioner's hand

↳ Painful during? Rarely

↳ Aims at: Joint motion and muscle tone

Chiropractic adjustment

↳ Force: A quick thrust to a joint

↳ Painful during? Brief discomfort possible

↳ Aims at: Joint position and motion

Dry needling

↳ Force: A thin needle into a trigger point

↳ Painful during? A brief twitch or ache is common

↳ Aims at: Trigger points in muscle

Physical therapy exercise

↳ Force: Your own effort

↳ Painful during? Can be, as load builds

↳ Aims at: Strength, mobility, and movement patterns

Strain-Counterstrain belongs to a family of methods often called positional release. If you see that term on a clinic's site, it's a close relative.

None of these rules out the others. Some people use two at once, and it's worth telling each practitioner what the other is doing.

Your Playbook

Copy this section and send it. It stands on its own, with no context from the rest of the book.

> **1.** Write your full injury and surgery timeline, oldest first, to bring to the appointment
>
> *Owner: You · Time: 20 min*

> **2.** Pick one repeatable movement and record your baseline the morning of the visit
>
> *Owner: You · Time: 5 min*

> **3.** Confirm the practitioner's training level when you book: Jones Institute courses completed, and whether they treat visceral and nervous system
>
> *Owner: You · Time: 5 min*

> **4.** Wear loose clothing. Block 90 minutes, not 45
>
> *Owner: You · Time: 0 min*

> **5.** Re-measure the same movement the next morning and again at 7 days
>
> *Owner: You · Time: 5 min*

The 3 rules that make it work.

1. **Say something if it hurts.** A correct technique is comfortable. Pain during treatment means the position is wrong.
2. **Bring the whole history.** The 1998 ankle sprain belongs on the list.
3. **Measure one thing objectively.** Pain memory shifts with the day you're having. A tape measure doesn't.

How you'll know it's working in 30 days. Your one measured movement has changed in a direction you can state in numbers, or it hasn't. Either answer is worth having.

After your first session, which one movement will tell you whether it worked?

PART TWO

What the Evidence Actually Says

CHAPTER 4

What Does the Research Show, and Where Is It Thin?

There's one randomized trial of Fascial Counterstrain, a set of small trials of its parent technique with mixed results, a published mechanism paper, and a set of case reports. The signal is real in places, the evidence base is small and early, and the Fascial Counterstrain work is mostly authored by people with a financial stake.

How much evidence would you want before trying something that carries almost no risk?

That question has a different answer than "how much evidence before surgery," and pretending otherwise is how people get talked out of low-risk options and into high-risk ones.

> ## Start Here: The 60-Second Version
>
> **The decision this chapter helps you make.**
> Whether the evidence justifies spending your money and a few hours on this, given what you've already spent.
>
> **The questions it answers.**
>
> ↳ What controlled trials exist, and what did they actually find?
>
> ↳ Who funded and authored them?

↳ Why isn't this in mainstream care if it works?

↳ What would change my mind, in either direction?

Why it matters. In the one randomized study of Fascial Counterstrain published to date, 22 analyzed participants with PTSD received either three 90-minute sessions or waitlist control. Clinician-rated symptom severity fell 18.7 points in the treatment group against 1.3 points in controls, with the difference between groups significant at $p = 0.0017$. That's a real result from a very small study run by people who sell the treatment. Both halves of that sentence are true and both matter.

What you walk away with. A clear map of what's known, what's claimed, and what's neither.

The strongest controlled evidence

Christy, Tuckey, Miljacic, Polissar, and Vythilingam. Military Medicine, published online August 2025, in print March 2026.

Twenty-four veterans and first responders with PTSD symptoms were randomized to Fascial Counterstrain or to a waitlist. Twenty-two were analyzed. The treatment group received three 90-minute sessions over an average of 19.5 days, using a protocol targeting the sympathetic nervous system.

The results, from the paper:

↳ Clinician-Administered PTSD Scale scores fell 18.7 points, 95% CI 8.7 to 28.7, against 1.3 points in the waitlist group.

↳ Every one of the 10 evaluable treated participants improved by at least one PTSD severity category. Two of 10 controls did.

↳ A clinically meaningful response, defined as a 10-point drop, occurred in 80% of the treatment group and 20% of controls, though that specific comparison reached only $p = 0.057$.

↳ Self-reported depression, anxiety, and somatic symptoms all improved significantly against controls.

↳ Improvement was sustained through 6 months of follow-up.

↳ No adverse events in either group.

The authors note the size of the effect was comparable to what's reported after 6 weeks of sertraline or 8 weeks of certain psychotherapies, and that it happened in about 20 days.

Now the limits, which the authors state themselves.

↳ It's a proof-of-concept study with 22 analyzed participants. That's small.

↳ The control was a waitlist, not an active comparator. Waitlist controls can inflate apparent effects, because only the treated group gets attention, expectation, and the simple act of being taken seriously.

- ↳ Participants couldn't be blinded. You know when someone has been manually treating you for 90 minutes.
- ↳ **The conflict of interest is substantial and disclosed.** Brian Tuckey developed Fascial Counterstrain, owns a clinic that provides it, and is a paid instructor for the organization that sells the training. Holly Christy owns a clinic that provides it and is also a paid instructor. Funding came from a nonprofit connected to the work.
- ↳ It studied PTSD, not chronic musculoskeletal pain, so it doesn't directly establish anything about your back.

That's a promising early signal from an interested party. It's the most rigorous thing this field has, and it's one small study.

The evidence for the parent technique

Koura and colleagues. Journal of Multidisciplinary Healthcare, January 2025.

Thirty adults with low back myofascial pain syndrome were randomized to Strain-Counterstrain plus standardized exercise, or standardized exercise alone, for 4 weeks.

- ↳ Pain fell 26.7% in the combined group against 5.2% in exercise alone.
- ↳ Oswestry Disability Index scores improved 25.2% against 2.3%.
- ↳ Lumbar range of motion improved more in the combined group across most directions.

↳ Both p values below 0.001.

The limits. Thirty participants across two arms is 15 each. The trial wasn't blinded. A methodological critique letter published in the same journal three weeks later flagged, among other issues, that the reported sample size calculation didn't reconcile with the stated effect size and power, and that the title described a comparison when both arms received exercise.

And the study tested Strain-Counterstrain, the original musculoskeletal method, not the Fascial Counterstrain expansion. Whoever hands you this study, it isn't proof of the visceral or vascular claims.

The trials that didn't find a difference. These matter just as much, and some are better designed.

↳ **Lewis and colleagues, Journal of Physiotherapy, 2011.** 89 adults with acute low back pain, with concealed allocation and a blinded assessor. Strain-Counterstrain plus exercise did no better than exercise alone at 2, 6, or 28 weeks. It's larger and more rigorous than the Koura trial.

↳ **Klein and colleagues, Complementary Therapies in Medicine, 2013.** 61 adults with neck pain. A single Strain-Counterstrain session did no better than a sham treatment on neck mobility or pain.

↳ **Segura-Ortí and colleagues, Acupuncture in Medicine, 2016.** 34 adults with neck trigger points. Strain-Counterstrain, dry needling, and sham Strain-Counterstrain all improved, with no difference between the groups.

What the reviews say. A 2014 meta-analysis of 5 trials found low-quality evidence that Strain-Counterstrain reduces tender-point pain. A 2025 systematic review of 18 positional release trials in low back pain, covering 918 people, found very low certainty of benefit when it's added to other treatment, and no benefit shown when it's used on its own. One of that review's authors works for a positional release training institute.

What does that add up to? Promising in places, mixed in others, and unproven overall, for a treatment that carries little risk. Most of these trials tested 1 to 4 short sessions of the original method, not the longer full-body Fascial Counterstrain protocol. That gap cuts both ways: these trials don't prove Fascial Counterstrain works, and they don't settle that it doesn't. It's a strong reason to measure your own results.

The mechanism papers

Tuckey and colleagues, Frontiers in Pain Research, 2021, proposes the impaired lymphatic drainage model described in Chapter 2. It's a theoretical review. It assembles physiology, it doesn't test a treatment.

Tuckey, International Journal of Osteopathic Medicine, December 2025, describes the methodology and how Fascial Counterstrain differs from its predecessor. The author declares ownership of the copyrights on the techniques described. That disclosure is appropriate and it's also the point:

this is the developer describing his own method in a journal, which is a legitimate contribution and isn't independent verification.

The case reports

There's a body of published case studies, including one on calcific shoulder tendinitis that hadn't resolved after arthroscopic decompression and six weeks of post-operative rehabilitation.

Case reports are useful for one thing: showing that something is possible and worth studying. They can't tell you how often it happens, because the cases that didn't work rarely get published.

Two papers published in 2026

Two papers published this year matter, and they cut in opposite directions on the question of independence.

An objective measurement, from an interested party. In March 2026, a case study in the journal Lymphatics used quantitative sensory testing to measure a single patient before and after treatment. Temporal summation of pain, which measures how much a nervous system amplifies repeated stimuli, and pressure pain threshold were both recorded. After treatment, wind-up in the affected S1 and S2 dermatomes had nearly normalized, and pressure pain thresholds improved substantially.

That matters, because it's the first published attempt to move a measurement that isn't a questionnaire. It's also one patient, with the developer of the technique as an author, and the authors say plainly that ethical approval was waived because a single case report isn't human-subjects research. One case is a starting point, not a finding.

An independent randomized pilot. In July 2026, a researcher at Masan University in Korea published a randomized pilot in the Journal of Manual and Manipulative Therapy comparing Strain-Counterstrain against another manual method in 20 healthy adults with latent upper trapezius trigger points. All participants completed it, no adverse events were reported, and it found no difference between the two techniques. The author says no conclusions about effectiveness can be drawn from it yet. The author declared no conflict of interest and no funding.

Like the older trials of the parent technique above, it has no financial connection to anyone selling the method. It's small, it's in healthy volunteers rather than pain patients, and it has no untreated control group. It's thin, and it's still worth knowing it's there.

One more thing worth quoting. The nonprofit that funded the PTSD trial states on its own website that Fascial Counterstrain isn't an approved treatment for PTSD, that it's considered experimental, and that more research is needed.

When the people funding the research say that out loud, it's worth taking them at their word. It's also why I trust that research more, not less.

What about the Tony Robbins endorsement?

A testimonial attributed to Tony Robbins, published on the Counterstrain training company's own website, describes results he calls miraculous at times. It's a large part of why some people have heard of this technique at all.

A public figure saying something helped them is a testimonial. Testimonials tell you nothing about how many people it didn't help, because the people it didn't help rarely get interviewed.

I'm not saying he's wrong. I'm saying his experience isn't data, mine isn't data, and neither is a glowing review on a book page. Data is the boring table in a trial with a control group in it.

If a clinic's website leads with celebrity names rather than with what they will measure at your second visit, that tells you something about the clinic.

Why this isn't in mainstream care yet

If this is the first you've heard of it, you're in good company. There are four structural reasons, none of which involve anyone failing at their job.

It's taught post-graduate, not in school. A licensed clinician has to seek it out, pay for multi-day courses, and then keep taking them. The Fascial Counterstrain curriculum alone spans six systems.

It's time-expensive per patient. Sessions run 60 to 90 minutes. Standard outpatient physical therapy economics, driven by reimbursement, push toward shorter visits and multiple patients per hour. A technique that requires a full hour of one clinician's undivided attention fits poorly into that model regardless of whether it works.

The trial base is thin, and funders follow trial bases. Drug and device makers have little to gain from proving that a hands-on technique works, so the large trial that would settle it hasn't been funded yet.

It has no distribution channel. There's no sales force. It spreads clinician to clinician and patient to patient, which is slow.

None of that is evidence it works. It just explains why not having heard of it isn't evidence it doesn't.

What would change my mind

I'd find any of these persuasive in the other direction:

- ↳ A randomized trial with an active comparator, such as sham manual contact, that showed no difference.
- ↳ A trial run by investigators with no financial connection to the technique that failed to replicate.
- ↳ Evidence of harm beyond transient soreness.

And I'd find these persuasive in favor:

- ↳ A trial of 200 or more with an active control, in musculoskeletal pain rather than PTSD.
- ↳ Independent replication by a group that doesn't teach or sell the method.
- ↳ Objective biomarkers moving, not just questionnaires.

For the parent technique, a few small sham-controlled trials of short protocols already point the skeptical way, and I take that seriously. For Fascial Counterstrain itself, neither set exists yet. The independent pilot above is a first step, and the sensory-testing case study is a first attempt at an objective measure. Both are far too small to settle anything. That's where the field is in 2026, and anyone calling it settled has gone past what's known.

Why I wrote this

I told you in the introduction that 20-year-old knee pain resolved for me after the first appointment, and that I only heard the name because a friend mentioned it.

That's one person's story, and I've just spent a chapter explaining why anecdotes don't settle anything. Mine doesn't either.

So why write a book on thin evidence instead of waiting? Because I carried that knee for 20 years without knowing this existed, and I'd rather the next person didn't have to. The technique is grounded in anatomy and physiology, not something unfalsifiable. The risk of trying it is one appointment.

And outside one famous testimonial, there's almost nothing out there written for the people living with this.

I don't know whether your pain will respond the way mine did. I can share what happened, and what is and isn't known, and let you decide for yourself.

So what do you do with that

That one is yours, and it turns on things a book can't see: your history, your diagnosis, and what you've already carried.

What I can do is set the facts side by side, honestly, and trust you with them.

The technique is non-invasive, uses no force, has no reported serious adverse events in the published literature, and produces a same-day signal that can be checked. The evidence behind it is early, small, and largely produced by people with a financial interest in it. Both of those are true at the same time, and the right thing is to say both.

Underneath every treatment decision, in every field, sit the same two questions. What does it cost to be wrong, and how quickly would you know?

- ↳ What would you want to see, and by when, to call something worth continuing?
- ↳ What would being wrong about this cost, next to being wrong about the other options in front of you?

↳ What's already in place for this, and what would show you it had stopped earning its spot?

Thoughtful people land in different places on those, and there's no single right answer waiting at the end of them.

Your Playbook

Copy this section and send it. It stands on its own, with no context from the rest of the book.

> **1.** Read the Military Medicine paper abstract yourself. It's open access
>
> *Owner: You · Time: 10 min*

> **2.** Note the conflict of interest statement in that paper before you weigh the result
>
> *Owner: You · Time: 2 min*

> **3.** Decide your own evidence threshold for a low-risk intervention versus a high-risk one
>
> *Owner: You · Time: 10 min*

> **4.** Set a stop rule before you book: how many sessions with no measurable change before you stop
>
> *Owner: You · Time: 5 min*

> **5.** Ask any practitioner what they would consider evidence their treatment isn't working for you
>
> *Owner: You · Time: 2 min*

The 3 rules that make it work.

1. **Ask for more proof when there's more at stake.** A surgery and a pair of hands don't deserve the same level of scrutiny.
2. **Read the disclosure before the result.** In this field, the author often owns the clinic.
3. **Set the stop rule first.** Deciding in advance when to walk away is what keeps a trial from becoming a subscription.

How you'll know it's working in 30 days. You've written down, in advance, the number of sessions and the measurable change that will decide this for you.

How would you know whether a treatment is aimed at your symptoms or at what's causing them?

CHAPTER 5

What Has It Been Used For, and What Is It Not For?

Practitioners report using it across musculoskeletal, nerve, vascular, lymphatic, and visceral complaints. The controlled evidence covers low back pain and PTSD. Everything else is clinical report, and the gap between those two sentences is where it pays to be careful.

Which of your symptoms have you been told are unrelated to each other?

> ### Start Here: The 60-Second Version
>
> **The decision this chapter helps you make.** Whether your specific situation is plausibly in scope, and when to go somewhere else instead.
>
> **The questions it answers.**
>
> ↳ What conditions do practitioners actually treat with this?
>
> ↳ Which of those claims have controlled evidence behind them?
>
> ↳ When is this the wrong answer, or a dangerous delay?

↳ How do I tell an honest practitioner from an over-reaching one?

Why it matters. The Fascial Counterstrain curriculum covers six anatomical systems, which is why the reported condition list runs from frozen shoulder to post-surgical abdominal pain. A wide scope of practice is a real feature and a real risk. It's why practitioners report reaching things other approaches hadn't, and why some clinics claim far more than the evidence supports.

What you walk away with. A clear line between what's reported, what's proven, and what should send you to a physician today.

What has actually been tested

Short list, and worth keeping in front of the longer one.

Chronic low back myofascial pain

↳ Evidence: One small randomized trial of the parent technique, favorable; a critique letter questioned its methods

↳ Source: Koura et al., 2025, n=30

Acute low back pain

↳ Evidence: The largest, most rigorous trial of the parent technique found no added benefit over exercise

↳ Source: Lewis et al., 2011, n=89

Low back pain of any type

↳ Evidence: Systematic review of positional release: very low certainty of benefit as an add-on, none shown on its own

↳ Source: Danazumi et al., 2025, 18 trials

Neck pain

↳ Evidence: A single session matched sham in one trial; added to standard therapy, it did better in another

↳ Source: Klein et al., 2013, n=61; El-Khateeb et al., 2022

Neck trigger points

↳ Evidence: No difference between the parent technique, dry needling, and sham

↳ Source: Segura-Ortí et al., 2016, n=34

Tension-type headache

↳ Evidence: Matched medication in one small trial and beat a control group in another

↳ Source: Ghanbari et al., 2012, n=30; Mohamadi et al., 2020, 26 analyzed

Plantar fasciitis

↳ Evidence: Small crossover trial against a placebo capsule; relief lasted about 48 hours

↳ Source: Wynne et al., 2006, n=20

Chronic ankle instability

↳ Evidence: Better balance than sham, with no difference in self-rated function

↳ Source: Collins et al., 2014, n=27

PTSD symptom severity

↳ Evidence: One small randomized trial of Fascial Counterstrain, waitlist control

↳ Source: Christy et al., 2025, n=22 analyzed

Everything else

↳ Evidence: Clinical report and case studies only

↳ Source: Various

That list is where things stand: promising in places, mixed in others. Most of it tested the parent technique, not Fascial Counterstrain, and it's more useful than a longer list that blurs the difference.

What practitioners report treating

This is the reported scope, offered as reported scope and nothing more.

Musculoskeletal. Low back and neck pain, frozen shoulder, hip and knee pain, plantar fasciitis, post-surgical stiffness, chronic tendinopathy.

Nervous system. Sciatica, carpal tunnel symptoms, thoracic outlet symptoms, migraine and cervicogenic headache, post-concussion symptoms, trigeminal pain.

Vascular and lymphatic. Persistent swelling, cold hands and feet, symptoms attributed to circulation in an extremity.

Visceral. Post-surgical abdominal and pelvic pain, including after C-section, hernia repair, and appendectomy. Chronic pelvic pain. Symptoms overlapping with irritable bowel syndrome (IBS).

Autonomic. Postural Orthostatic Tachycardia Syndrome (POTS) and other dysautonomia symptoms, including post-viral presentations.

Central sensitization. Widespread pain presentations, including fibromyalgia, are what the newer Central Sensitization Series was built for. Chapter 8 covers the strongest non-drug trial in fibromyalgia, which tested tai chi.

The autonomic and visceral claims are the ones to hold most loosely. They're also, interestingly, where the one randomized FCS trial happens to point, since the protocol in that study targeted the sympathetic nervous system.

An illustrative example

About this example. The following is an illustrative composite drawn from patterns commonly described in this work, not a specific patient. Details are invented. It's here to show the reasoning, not to serve as evidence.

A runner presents with knee pain of three years. Imaging is unremarkable. Physical therapy strengthened her quadriceps and glutes, which helped for a month at a time, twice.

A practitioner working from this model takes her history and finds an ankle fracture at 19 with six weeks in a cast, and a laparoscopic appendectomy at 31. Her scan finds tender points along the same-side lower abdomen and hip.

The hypothesis is that the pain generator isn't the knee, and the knee is where a longstanding alteration in how she loads that leg finally became symptomatic.

That's a testable hypothesis. Within two sessions she either has more pain-free running distance or she doesn't. That's the part worth copying, whatever your condition is: a named tissue, and a short timeline to be wrong.

Can a C-section or old surgery cause pain years later?

About this example. An illustrative composite drawn from patterns commonly described in this work, not a specific patient. Details are invented.

A mother of two has had a pulling pain low in her abdomen since an emergency C-section 5 years ago. The scar looks fine and her scans are normal. A practitioner working from this model checks the tissue around the scar, not only where it hurts. The testable version: does standing fully upright, or lifting her youngest, feel different within 2 sessions?

What about POTS, or dizziness after a virus?

About this example. An illustrative composite drawn from patterns commonly described in this work, not a specific patient. Details are invented.

Months after a viral illness, a woman in her 30s gets lightheaded and her heart races when she stands. Her tilt-table test points to POTS. Practitioners report treating presentations like this, and it's the claim in this book to hold most loosely: it rests on clinical report alone. The testable version: how long can she stand before symptoms start, measured the morning of a session and again a week later?

When this is the wrong answer

Go to a physician, not a manual therapist, if you have:

↳ New or progressive weakness, numbness, or loss of coordination

↳ Numbness in the groin or saddle area, or any change in bladder or bowel control

↳ Fever with back pain, or pain that's dramatically worse at night and unrelieved by position

↳ Unexplained weight loss, or a personal history of cancer

↳ Pain after significant trauma, or any suspicion of fracture

↳ Chest pain, shortness of breath, or new severe headache

↳ Signs of infection over the area

Counterstrain is also not the answer for an acute fracture, an active infection, an unstable joint, an untreated blood clot, or a condition where a delay in diagnosis is what harms you.

A responsible practitioner screens for these and refers out. If a practitioner tells you they can treat something that clearly belongs to a physician, that's a signal to look elsewhere.

How to tell an honest practitioner from an overreaching one

Five signals, and none of them require you to know anatomy.

They name a tissue and a timeline. Chapter 1's question. An honest answer is specific and falsifiable.

They recheck in front of you. Palpate, treat, palpate again, tell you what changed. If nobody ever rechecks, nobody is testing anything.

They tell you when to stop. "If you haven't seen a change by session 3, this isn't your answer" is one of the most trust-earning sentences in this field.

They don't sell packages up front. Pre-paid blocks of 12 visits are a business model, not a treatment plan.

They say "I don't know." Anyone who can treat everything is treating nothing in particular.

Your Playbook

Copy this section and send it. It stands on its own, with no context from the rest of the book.

> **1.** Check your symptoms against the red flag list above before doing anything else
>
> *Owner: You · Time: 5 min*

> **2.** If any red flag is present, book a physician appointment this week
>
> *Owner: You · Time: 10 min*

> **3.** List every symptom you have, including the ones that seem unrelated to the pain
>
> *Owner: You · Time: 10 min*

> **4.** Ask the practitioner which of your symptoms they expect to change and which they don't
>
> *Owner: You · Time: 5 min*

> **5.** Write down their answer. Compare it to what actually happens
>
> *Owner: You · Time: 2 min*

The 3 rules that make it work.

1. **Red flags outrank everything in this book.** Always.

2. **What practitioners treat and what's been tested are two different lists.** Hold the visceral and autonomic claims the most loosely.
3. **"I don't know" is a green flag.** Certainty about everything is the warning sign.

How you'll know it's working in 30 days. You have a written prediction from your practitioner about which symptoms should move, and you can check it against reality.

Which of your symptoms has cost you the most, and what would you do differently if it were resolved?

PART THREE

Getting Care Without Wasting Money

CHAPTER 6

How Do I Find a Practitioner and Not Waste the First Session?

Use the Jones Institute and Counterstrain Academy directories, check which courses the practitioner has completed, and arrive with a written timeline and one measured movement.

How many first appointments have you spent re-explaining your history from memory?

> ### Start Here: The 60-Second Version
>
> **The decision this chapter helps you make.** Who to book with, and what to bring so the first hour counts.
>
> **The questions it answers.**
>
> ↳ Where do I actually find someone trained in this?
>
> ↳ What do the credentials mean, and which ones matter?
>
> ↳ What should I prepare before I walk in?
>
> ↳ What questions should I ask before I hand over a card?
>
> **Why it matters.** Counterstrain training is post-graduate and modular, so two practitioners with the same li-

> cense can have very different scope. The Fascial Counterstrain curriculum covers over 900 techniques across six anatomical systems, and clinicians take those courses one at a time over years. Asking which ones someone has completed is one of the highest-value questions you can ask before booking.
>
> **What you walk away with.** A shortlist, a prepared history, and a baseline measurement.

Where to look

The Jones Institute practitioner directory is the primary source, since the Jones Institute runs the foundational courses. Their patient-facing directory is at jicounterstrain.configio.com/accountdirectory.

The Counterstrain Academy clinic finder at academy.counterstrain.com/clinics lists clinics whose practitioners have gone through the mastery program.

Ask your existing physical therapist. Some DPTs have taken these courses without advertising it, because it's one tool among many in their practice. It costs you one question.

Access is genuinely uneven. In some metro areas you'll find several options. In rural areas you may find none within a reasonable drive, and telehealth isn't an option for a hands-on technique. If that's your situation, Chapters 8 and 9 exist for you specifically.

What the credentials mean

Worth understanding, because the letters aren't self-explanatory.

A state license is the floor. The Jones Institute requires a state-issued healthcare license to register for its courses, because the curriculum assumes advanced anatomy and physiology. Physical therapists, occupational therapists, massage therapists, osteopathic physicians, athletic trainers, chiropractors, and other licensed clinicians are all eligible.

SCS versus FCS. Ask which they have. Strain-Counterstrain covers roughly 200 musculoskeletal techniques. Fascial Counterstrain adds over 900 across six systems and is what you want if your issue is visceral, vascular, or autonomic.

Which FCS systems. This is the question that gets asked least and matters most. The FCS courses are separate: Foundations first, then Musculoskeletal, Lymphatic-Venous, Arterial, Visceral, Nervous System, plus a central sensitization series. Someone who has taken Foundations and Musculoskeletal is well trained and can't treat post-surgical abdominal pain. It's worth asking.

JSCCI means Jones Strain Counterstrain Certified Instructor, which is the teaching credential. **Board certification** in Jones Strain Counterstrain requires passing an exam. Both signal depth. Neither is required for someone to be good.

Counterstrain Academy mastery program. A separate post-course mentorship track with its own modules, each requiring the matching Jones Institute course as a prerequisite. Practitioners in or through this program have gone well past the minimum.

What to bring

A written timeline, oldest first. Every fracture, sprain, surgery, car accident, fall from a height, childbirth, concussion, and significant illness with approximate dates. Yes, including the ones from childhood. Yes, including the ones nobody has ever asked about.

It's one of the highest-leverage things you can do. A practitioner working from this model is looking for where the fascial history starts, and you're the only person who has that information.

A symptom list, including the ones you think are unrelated. Bloating, dizziness on standing, cold hands, headaches, swelling, sleep problems. They don't have to seem connected. Writing them down is enough.

Your baseline measurement. The one repeatable movement from Chapter 3, recorded that morning.

Your imaging reports, if you've got them. The report is more useful than the images.

Your stop rule. It's in Chapter 7. Decide it before you go, not after session 4. A printable version of the timeline, the 5 questions below, and a stop-rule line is free at LeadWithGold.com/first-visit-kit.

What to ask before you book

Five questions, by phone or email, in under three minutes.

1. Which Jones Institute courses have you completed, and do you treat the visceral and nervous systems?
2. How long is a first session, and how long is a follow-up?
3. What's the cost per session, and do you bill insurance or provide a superbill?
4. How many sessions before we'd know whether this is helping me?
5. What would tell you this isn't the right treatment for my case?

Question 5 is the one that sorts the field. Anyone who can answer it well has thought about being wrong, and that's the practitioner worth booking.

What the scan is for

Practitioners describe one pattern that shortens a first session more than anything else: the appointment stays on the painful area, because that's the area everyone came in thinking about.

Which is completely natural. It's also the one thing the scan exists to get past.

If the model in this chapter holds for a given case, the cause can sit somewhere that's hard to guess, and the whole reason for scanning the body rather than the complaint is to let it turn up. A session steered toward the right shoulder becomes a session about the right shoulder.

Your Playbook

Copy this section and send it. It stands on its own, with no context from the rest of the book.

> **1.** Search the Jones Institute directory and the Counterstrain Academy clinic finder for your area
>
> *Owner: You · Time: 15 min*

> **2.** Email or call 2 practitioners with the 5 questions above
>
> *Owner: You · Time: 15 min*

> **3.** Write your full injury, surgery, and illness timeline, oldest first
>
> *Owner: You · Time: 25 min*

> **4.** Write your symptom list, including symptoms you believe are unrelated
>
> *Owner: You · Time: 10 min*

> **5.** Record your baseline movement measurement the morning of the appointment
>
> *Owner: You · Time: 5 min*

> **6.** Write down your stop rule and put it in your phone
> *Owner: You · Time: 5 min*

The 3 rules that make it work.

1. **Ask which systems they trained in.** Same license, very different scope.
2. **The timeline is your job.** Nobody else has it, and it's the input the whole method runs on.
3. **Decide your stop rule before the first visit.** Not after the fourth.

How you'll know it's working in 30 days. You've booked with someone whose training matches your problem, and you walked in with a written history instead of trying to remember it under pressure.

What's in your history that nobody has ever asked you about?

CHAPTER 7

How Many Sessions, What Does It Cost, and When Do I Stop?

Fewer than most people expect. The work is built around resolving what's driving the pain rather than managing it, so the aim is to finish. Practitioners commonly describe a handful of sessions. That figure comes from clinics that provide the treatment, and the one randomized study used three.

What has managing this cost you so far, counting the parts that never showed up on a bill?

> ### Start Here: The 60-Second Version
>
> **The decision this chapter helps you make.** How much to commit before you decide, and when to stop.
>
> **The questions it answers.**
>
> ↳ How many sessions does this actually take?
>
> ↳ What does it cost and will insurance cover it?
>
> ↳ How do I avoid this turning into another open-ended subscription?
>
> ↳ What does "no maintenance needed" actually mean?

> **Why it matters.** The one randomized Fascial Counterstrain study delivered three 90-minute sessions over an average of 19.5 days and measured sustained change at 6 months. That's the only session count with a control group attached to it. Every other number you'll hear, including the one in this technique's own marketing, comes from clinics reporting on their own patients.
>
> **What you walk away with.** A budget, a stop rule, and language for the conversation with your practitioner.

What you'll hear, and how much weight to give it

The figure circulated most often in this field is that most people's primary complaints resolve in roughly 1 to 6 sessions, with more complex histories taking longer.

Where that comes from. Clinic-reported experience. It isn't a trial result and it isn't from an independent source. It's a group of people who provide a treatment describing how their own patients do.

That doesn't make it false. Clinicians usually have a decent sense of their own outcomes. It does mean it sits closer to an expectation than to a finding, and it's the kind of number that can be tested on one person rather than believed or disbelieved.

What the controlled data says. Three 90-minute sessions produced a measurable, sustained effect in one small randomized study of PTSD symptoms. That's it. That's the whole controlled dataset on dose.

What it costs

Prices are set by individual clinics and vary widely by region and by practitioner. Ask directly. Typical structures you'll encounter:

- ↳ **First session**, usually 60 to 90 minutes, priced higher than follow-ups.
- ↳ **Follow-up sessions**, often 45 to 60 minutes.
- ↳ **Cash-pay is common**, particularly for practitioners whose visits run long, because standard reimbursement doesn't fund a 90-minute one-on-one appointment well.

On insurance. Many practitioners are physical therapists, and the visit may be billable as physical therapy using standard manual therapy codes even though the specific technique isn't separately recognized. Others are out of network and provide a superbill you submit yourself.

Two things to ask before you book:

1. Do you bill my insurance, or do you provide a superbill?
2. If you bill insurance, does my plan require a physician referral or a visit limit?

Health savings and flexible spending accounts generally cover physical therapy from a licensed provider. Confirm with your administrator rather than assuming, and keep the receipt.

The number most people have never added up

There's a figure that almost never gets seen in chronic pain, because it never arrives as a single bill.

Copays. Massage. Chiropractic. Over-the-counter medication. Braces and supports. Injections. Imaging. Days off work. Spread across 12 months, none of it lands together, so there's nothing sitting in one place to look at.

↳ What did the last 12 months of managing this add up to?

↳ Which parts of it arrived in pieces small enough to disappear into an ordinary month?

↳ What would you want that figure to be next year?

Those answers belong to you, and nobody else needs to see them. They're here because it's natural to weigh any new cost against zero, and managing this has been costing something all along.

How to keep this from becoming a subscription

This is the part where people get hurt financially, and it applies to every therapy, not just this one.

Decide the stop rule before session one. A reasonable default: if nothing measurable has changed after 3 sessions, stop and reassess. Not "I feel about the same." Measurable. Your movement test from Chapter 3.

A pre-paid package before a first visit is worth a pause. A practitioner who needs 12 sessions up front has told you their business model, not their clinical judgment.

Ask what "done" looks like. At session one, ask: what does discharge look like, and how will we know when we're there? A treatment model built on resolving something rather than managing it should be able to describe its own endpoint.

Watch for goalpost drift. If the target keeps moving from your back, to your posture, to your general wellness, without your original complaint changing, that's your signal.

Managing it and resolving it are two different goals

This is the part that made me want to write the book, so I'll be plain about it.

If a sweater keeps snagging on the same nail, you can keep mending the sweater. Or you can find the nail.

Most of what's offered for chronic pain is built around management. Come back weekly. Keep up the exercises. Take the medication. Those things can help, and a plan built on management has no finish line in it by design.

The claim underneath Counterstrain is different. It's that a specific restriction, once released, stays released unless something new re-establishes it. Not suppressed, not managed. Released. So the goal of the work is to run out of things to treat.

That's why practitioners talk in terms of a handful of sessions rather than a standing appointment, and why the question to ask any practitioner is what discharge looks like.

What that means in practice. You're not signing up for something indefinite. You're testing a hypothesis about the cause, and a hypothesis fails fast and cheap or it resolves something.

What it doesn't mean. It doesn't make anyone immune. A new injury, a surgery, or a significant illness can create new restrictions, and people do come back years later for something new. That's a different problem, not a relapse.

What hasn't been formally measured. There's no long-term controlled follow-up in musculoskeletal pain. The PTSD study followed people for 6 months and the effect held, which is the longest controlled follow-up this technique has, and it's in a different condition than yours.

So this is where it stands. The model is built around resolution rather than maintenance, practitioners consistently report it behaves that way, one small study showed a 6-month hold in a different condition, and durability in chronic musculoskeletal pain hasn't been formally studied yet. Anyone promising permanence has gone past what's known.

What none of that changes is the goal. The point of finding a cause is to be done with it.

What helps between sessions?

Can you do Counterstrain on yourself? Partly, and carefully. A physician-written self-help adaptation exists, Dale Anderson's *Muscle Pain Relief in 90 Seconds*, built on the same fold-and-hold idea for muscles. No controlled trial has tested self-applied Counterstrain. The visceral, vascular, and nervous-system work isn't something a person can do on themselves, and a practitioner who knows your case is the right person to ask whether a home position suits it.

Does staying active help more than resting? For acute low back pain, a Cochrane review found advice to stay active did slightly better than advice to rest in bed. The difference is small, and it points the same direction as most of this book.

Is a flare the same as damage? Not necessarily. Pain after a busy day can be a flare rather than new harm, especially when it settles within a day or two. New numbness or weakness is different, and it's a reason to call a clinician.

What keeps it honest? The one movement from Chapter 3, measured at the same time of day. The next-morning number tends to tell you more than a same-day test of the area that was just treated.

What costs nothing? Walking, slow breathing, and the other free options in Chapter 8 sit comfortably alongside hands-on care.

Your Playbook

Copy this section and send it. It stands on its own, with no context from the rest of the book.

> **1.** Add up what you spent on this problem last year, including time off work
>
> *Owner: You · Time: 20 min*

> **2.** Get per-session pricing and the insurance or superbill answer in writing before booking
>
> *Owner: You · Time: 10 min*

> **3.** Confirm HSA or FSA eligibility with your plan administrator
>
> *Owner: You · Time: 10 min*

> **4.** Write your stop rule: number of sessions, and the measurable change required
>
> *Owner: You · Time: 5 min*

> **5.** At session 1, ask what discharge looks like and write down the answer
>
> *Owner: You · Time: 2 min*

> **6.** Decline any pre-paid package offered before you've had one session
>
> *Owner: You · Time: 0 min*

The 3 rules that make it work.

1. **Your stop rule needs a number in it, not a feeling.** "About the same" isn't a measurement.
2. **Don't pre-pay a block before session one.** The same goes for any therapy.
3. **Ask what done looks like.** A model built on resolution can describe its own finish line.

How you'll know it's working in 30 days. You know your annual spend on this problem, you've got a written stop rule, and you haven't pre-paid anything.

If you never had to spend another dollar managing this, what would you put that money toward instead?

PART FOUR

Beyond Counterstrain

CHAPTER 8

What Else Has Real Evidence That I Can Start Without a Practitioner?

Four things clear the bar of a randomized controlled trial in chronic pain: graded movement, tai chi, mindfulness-based stress reduction, and pain reprocessing therapy. One costs nothing, and free versions exist for two more. One popular routine you may have been told about has no controlled evidence at all, and this chapter says which.

What would you be willing to start this week, if it were free and took ten minutes a day?

Start Here: The 60-Second Version

The decision this chapter helps you make. What to start this week while you wait for an appointment, or instead of one if no practitioner is within reach.

The questions it answers.

↳ Which self-directed approaches have randomized trial evidence?

↳ What do the Five Tibetan Rites actually have behind them?

↳ Is there anything that has produced pain-free outcomes rather than just less pain?

> ↳ What can my employer already be covering that I don't know about?
>
> **Why it matters.** In a randomized trial of 151 adults with chronic back pain published in JAMA Psychiatry in 2022, 66% of participants assigned to pain reprocessing therapy were pain-free or nearly pain-free after 4 weeks, against 20% assigned to open-label placebo and 10% assigned to usual care. Participants averaged 10 years of pain before the trial. Effect sizes were larger than what's typically seen in chronic pain research.
>
> **What you walk away with.** Four evidence-backed options ranked by what they cost you, and one correction.

First, about the Five Tibetan Rites

I'm asked about this routine often, so here's what I found when I went looking.

What it is. A sequence of 5 repeated movements: a spin, a supine leg raise, a kneeling backbend, a tabletop or reverse plank, and a downward-to-upward dog transition. It comes from a 1939 book, and the health claims attached to it have always come from that book and from practitioner report.

What the research says. I searched for randomized controlled trials of the Five Tibetan Rites specifically. There aren't any worth reporting. Not a thin evidence base, not a mixed evidence base. The controlled literature on this specific named protocol is effectively empty.

What that does and doesn't mean. It doesn't mean the movements are worthless. Five minutes of daily mobility and spinal movement is a good thing, and if you enjoy this sequence and it gets you moving, keep doing it. You're almost certainly getting the well-established benefits of regular movement.

It does mean the routine hasn't been shown to do what the options below have been shown to do. It can sit alongside them. It can't yet stand in for them.

The four with real trials behind them

1. Movement, at a dose you can actually sustain

This is the least glamorous and best-supported item on the list.

For chronic low back pain, exercise therapy is a first-line recommendation across major clinical guidelines, and the finding that matters most is unromantic: **no single type of exercise is clearly superior.** Walking, swimming, resistance training, and Pilates all produce similar modest improvements. The type that works is the type you'll still be doing in 12 weeks.

Cost. Free.

How to start. Pick the smallest daily amount you're confident you can hold for a month. If that's a 10-minute walk, that's the right dose. Increasing too fast is a common reason people stop.

The reframe worth having. Hurting during movement and being damaged by movement aren't the same thing. In chronic primary pain, graded exposure to movement is the treatment, not a risk to be managed. A clinician who knows your case should confirm that applies to you.

2. Tai chi, particularly for fibromyalgia

The evidence. Wang and colleagues, BMJ, 2018. A 52-week randomized trial of 226 adults with fibromyalgia compared supervised aerobic exercise twice weekly for 24 weeks against four tai chi arms of varying dose.

Tai chi at the same dose as the exercise group produced a 16.2-point greater improvement on the Revised Fibromyalgia Impact Questionnaire, 95% CI 8.7 to 23.6, $p < 0.001$. Participants attended tai chi sessions more often than they attended aerobic exercise. No serious adverse events were related to either intervention.

Aerobic exercise is a standard non-drug recommendation for fibromyalgia. This trial found a mind-body practice matched or beat it.

Cost. Community classes are inexpensive. Free instruction exists online, though the trial used supervised in-person classes and that distinction is real.

Who it fits. Anyone with widespread pain, fatigue, and poor sleep. Also anyone for whom exercise programs haven't stuck, because the adherence finding in that trial isn't a footnote.

3. Mindfulness-based stress reduction

The evidence. Cherkin and colleagues, JAMA, 2016. A randomized trial of 342 adults aged 20 to 70 with chronic low back pain, average 7.3 years of pain, comparing mindfulness-based stress reduction (MBSR), cognitive behavioral therapy (CBT), and usual care. MBSR and CBT were delivered in eight weekly 2-hour groups.

At 26 weeks, clinically meaningful improvement in functional limitation occurred in 60.5% of the MBSR group and 57.7% of the CBT group, against 44.1% for usual care. Clinically meaningful improvement in pain bothersomeness occurred in 43.6% of MBSR and 44.9% of CBT, against 26.6% for usual care. The MBSR benefit held at 52 weeks.

Two notes. The effects were moderate, which is typical for chronic back pain treatments. And they were achieved even though only about half of those assigned to MBSR attended at least 6 of the 8 sessions, which tells you something encouraging about the dose required.

Cost. Standard 8-week MBSR courses are widely available, often through hospital systems, and free or low-cost versions exist. Some employer plans cover them.

4. Pain reprocessing therapy: what is it, and does it work?

This is the strongest single result in this chapter and the least known.

The evidence. Ashar and colleagues, JAMA Psychiatry, 2022. A randomized trial of 151 adults with chronic back pain, averaging 10 years of pain, assigned to 4 weeks of pain reprocessing therapy, open-label placebo injection, or usual care.

Of those assigned to the therapy, 33 of 50, or 66%, reported a pain intensity of 0 or 1 out of 10 at the end of treatment. In the placebo group it was 10 of 51, or 20%. In usual care, 5 of 50, or 10%. Gains were largely maintained at 1-year follow-up.

Functional MRI showed reduced prefrontal responses to evoked back pain in the treated group. The effect on pain was statistically mediated by reduced belief that the pain indicated tissue damage.

What it is. A structured psychological treatment that works on how the brain classifies the pain signal. That doesn't make the pain imaginary. The signal is real, and so is the pain. It targets primary chronic pain, meaning pain where no ongoing peripheral cause has been identified, which is roughly 85% of chronic back pain cases.

The limits. It was tested in people with low-to-moderate severity primary chronic back pain, not in people with an identified structural cause. A published critique in the same journal argued the control conditions weren't well matched. And several authors have commercial relationships with pain treatment companies, which is disclosed in the paper.

Cost. It requires a trained therapist, which is the barrier. Books describing the approach exist. The trial delivered nine sessions over 4 weeks. The Pain Reprocessing Therapy Institute, which trains practitioners in the method, keeps a practitioner directory at painreprocessingtherapy.com.

The one that sits somewhere between home and a clinic

Disclosure. As the Disclosure at the front of this book notes, my business can arrange access to programs like this one through employers, so I have a financial interest in this section. Everything below is held to the same evidence standard as the rest of the book.

What it is. Remote musculoskeletal care programs pair you with a licensed physical therapist and use computer vision through a phone or tablet to give real-time feedback on your form during home exercise. You do the sessions at home, on your schedule, with a human clinician overseeing the plan.

What the independent reviewer found. The Peterson Health Technology Institute evaluates health technology and sells none of it. In June 2024 it found that therapist-guided remote programs improve pain and function about as well as in-person physical therapy, with lower total spending. App-only programs without a therapist weren't found to be a full substitute.

What the trials found. Two randomized trials, in chronic back pain and chronic shoulder pain, compared therapist-guided remote programs with in-person physical therapy. Neither found a meaningful difference on the main outcome, and in the back pain trial fewer people dropped out: 15.7% against 34.3%. Both were sponsored by the company whose program was tested. Separately, a 12-month trial of 1,237 people in Germany found pain fell 46% on a digital care pathway, against 24% with standard care.

What brochures tend to leave out. Headline figures of 60% to 80% pain reduction usually come from people who finished a program, with no comparison group. People who quit aren't counted, which inflates the result. A widely cited 58% lower rate of surgery comes from a company-funded look back at records, not a randomized trial.

So the accurate version. About as good as in-person physical therapy, better than standard care, and done at home. That matters most when the nearest practitioner is an hour away, or weekday appointments aren't realistic.

How to get it. It's usually an employer or health plan benefit, not a retail purchase. Many people have one available without knowing it. Benefits emails get buried, so a benefits portal can be worth a look.

How to choose among these

Ranked by cost to you, lowest first.

Daily movement at a sustainable dose

↳ Cost: Free

↳ Evidence: Guideline-level, no type superior

↳ Best fit: Almost anyone. Start here

Slow-paced breathing (Chapter 9)

↳ Cost: Free

↳ Evidence: Consistent physiological effect

↳ Best fit: Anyone, especially with stress-linked flares

Tai chi

↳ Cost: Low

↳ Evidence: BMJ 2018, n=226

↳ Best fit: Fibromyalgia, widespread pain, poor adherence to exercise

MBSR

↳ Cost: Low to moderate

↳ Evidence: JAMA 2016, n=342

↳ Best fit: Chronic low back pain, high stress load

Pain reprocessing therapy

↳ Cost: Moderate, needs a therapist

↳ Evidence: JAMA Psychiatry 2022, n=151

↳ Best fit: Primary chronic pain, normal imaging, pain that moves or tracks stress

Remote musculoskeletal program

↳ Cost: Employer benefit

↳ Evidence: Independent assessment plus 2 RCTs showing equivalence

↳ Best fit: No local practitioner, no weekday hours

Every trial above tested one thing at a time, which is worth knowing when four of them look appealing at once. Running one of them properly tends to tell you more than spreading across four.

So the useful question isn't which one sounds best. It's which one you'd still be doing in a month.

Your Playbook

Copy this section and send it. It stands on its own, with no context from the rest of the book.

> **1.** Pick the smallest daily movement dose you're confident you can hold for 30 days
>
> *Owner: You · Time: 10 min*

> **2.** Search for a community tai chi class or an MBSR course through a local hospital system
>
> *Owner: You · Time: 20 min*

3. If your imaging is normal and your pain moves or tracks stress, read about pain reprocessing therapy

Owner: You · Time: 30 min

4. Check your employer benefits portal for a virtual musculoskeletal or physical therapy benefit

Owner: You · Time: 10 min

5. Choose exactly one to start. Write the start date down

Owner: You · Time: 5 min

6. Re-measure your one movement from Chapter 3 at 30 days

Owner: You · Time: 5 min

The 3 rules that make it work.

1. **One at a time.** You can't tell what worked if you started four things on Monday.
2. **The one you'll keep doing beats the better one you won't.** A 10-minute walk you actually take beats a program you abandon in week 2.
3. **Lots of people doing something isn't the same as it having been tested.** Ask what the trial was before you credit the routine.

How you'll know it's working in 30 days. You've done one chosen practice on at least 20 of 30 days, and you've got a before-and-after number for your one movement.

If the energy this takes from you came back, what would you spend it on?

CHAPTER 9

Does How You Breathe Actually Change Your Pain?

Slow breathing at roughly 5.5 to 6 breaths per minute reliably shifts autonomic balance and increases heart rate variability, and that effect is well replicated. Several of the more viral breathing practices aren't supported, and one of them carries a real safety risk.

Can changing how you breathe actually reduce pain, or is that wishful thinking?

Start Here: The 60-Second Version

The decision this chapter helps you make. Whether to spend 10 minutes a day on breathing practice, and which practices to avoid.

The questions it answers.

- ↳ What's actually established about breathing and the nervous system?
- ↳ Which breathing claims hold up, and which don't?
- ↳ What's the simplest protocol that has evidence behind it?

Why it matters. Breathing at about 6 breaths per minute produces maximal increases in heart rate variability and improves baroreflex sensitivity, an effect ordinary breathing at typical rates doesn't produce. That's one of the more consistently replicated findings in this area, and the intervention is free.

What you walk away with. A 10-minute practice you can start tonight, for free.

Why a chapter on breathing in a book about fascia

Because chronic pain and the autonomic nervous system are linked in both directions, and breathing is the one autonomic input you can operate on deliberately.

Chapter 4 described the one randomized Fascial Counterstrain trial, whose entire protocol targeted the sympathetic nervous system. The same target is reachable, partially and for free, by changing your respiratory rate.

That isn't a claim that breathing replaces treatment. It's a claim that the cheapest lever available to you pulls on the same system.

What holds up from the popular breathing books

Nestor's 2020 book Breath brought nasal and slow breathing to a mainstream audience, and a lot of people found real benefit through it. It's also journalism rather than research, built from interviews, self-experiments, and historical accounts. Some of what it popularized is well supported. Some of it isn't, and the book doesn't always mark the difference.

The split, claim by claim:

Well supported: slow breathing shifts autonomic balance. The resonance frequency finding, that breathing at roughly 5.5 to 6 breaths per minute maximizes heart rate variability and improves baroreflex sensitivity, is replicated across many studies. Nestor calls this the perfect breath. The physiology is real and it isn't his claim, it predates the book by decades.

Well supported: paced breathing helps stress and anxiety outcomes. A systematic review of clinical trials of isolated breathing interventions with stress or anxiety outcomes found the majority of interventions produced improvement.

Supported, with a narrower scope than the book implies: nasal breathing. Nasal breathing filters, warms, and humidifies air, and adds resistance that slows the breath. Those are real. The stronger claims about athletic performance and broad disease prevention are thinner than the confident tone suggests.

Not established: the broad claims about skull and airway remodeling in adults. Interesting, under-evidenced, and not something to act on.

Breath is a good read. The slow breathing is the part with trials behind it. The rest is still waiting on them.

The breathing that actually has research behind it

Ten minutes. No equipment. No app required, though a paced-breathing app makes it easier.

Rate. Roughly 5.5 to 6 breaths per minute. That's a 5-second inhale and a 5-second exhale, or 5.5 and 5.5, depending on what feels sustainable.

Route. Through the nose, in and out, if your nose is clear.

Shape. Into the belly, not the upper chest. Put a hand below your navel and let it be the thing that moves.

Position. Sitting or lying. Not driving.

Duration. Start at 5 minutes, build to 10. Daily beats long.

A refinement with support. Making the exhale longer than the inhale increases vagally mediated heart rate variability. A 4-second inhale and a 6-second exhale gets you both the slow rate and the longer exhale.

What to expect. This isn't dramatic. You may feel calmer, you may not notice much on day one. The physiological effect is measurable whether or not it's remarkable to experience, and the reason to do it daily is cumulative, not acute.

When it helps most. If your pain reliably worsens on high-stress days, or if you're the person whose shoulders are already at your ears by 10 a.m., this is aimed directly at you.

What to avoid, and who should check first

Avoid breath-hold practices in or near water. Hyperventilation followed by breath-holding can cause loss of consciousness without warning. People have drowned this way. Never do these practices in a pool, a bath, or open water.

Avoid intensive hyperventilation-based methods without clearance if you've got uncontrolled high blood pressure, a cardiac arrhythmia, a seizure disorder, a history of fainting, glaucoma, or if you're pregnant. Slow-paced breathing at 5.5 to 6 breaths per minute is gentle and low risk. Cyclic hyperventilation protocols are a different thing with a different risk profile.

Stop if you get dizzy, tingly, or lightheaded. That's overbreathing, not progress. Return to a normal rate.

Don't use breathing practice to replace treatment for a diagnosed respiratory or cardiac condition. Talk to the clinician managing it.

Your Playbook

Copy this section and send it. It stands on its own, with no context from the rest of the book.

> **1.** Check whether you can breathe comfortably through your nose while awake. If not, see a physician before anything else
>
> *Owner: You · Time: 5 min*

> **2.** Set a daily 5-minute slot. Same time, tied to something you already do
>
> *Owner: You · Time: 5 min*

> **3.** Breathe at 5 seconds in, 5 seconds out, through the nose, belly moving
>
> *Owner: You · Time: 5 min / day*

> **4.** After a week, extend to 10 minutes and shift to 4 in, 6 out
>
> *Owner: You · Time: 10 min / day*

> **5.** Track pain on high-stress days before and after 30 days of practice
>
> *Owner: You · Time: 1 min / day*

The 3 rules that make it work.

1. **The speed is what does the work.** 5.5 to 6 breaths per minute is the number that matters.
2. **A little most days beats a lot once a week.** Ten minutes a day, not an hour on Sunday.
3. **Never breath-hold near water.** This one has killed people.

How you'll know it's working in 30 days. You've practiced on at least 20 of 30 days, and you can compare your pain on stressful days now against your notes from week 1.

When in your day does your breathing get shallow, and what's usually going on at that moment?

CHAPTER 10

What If I Want to Learn This and Treat People?

Counterstrain training is post-graduate continuing education for licensed clinicians. A state healthcare license is the entry requirement, the courses run as 3-day immersions, and the full Fascial Counterstrain curriculum is a multi-year commitment taken one system at a time.

What would change in your practice if you had something more to offer the patients still looking for an answer?

Start Here: The 60-Second Version

The decision this chapter helps you make.
Whether to pursue this training, and in what order.

The questions it answers.

↳ Who is eligible to train?

↳ What's the actual course sequence and how long does it take?

↳ What do the certifications mean and do I need one?

↳ What should I expect this to do to my practice model?

> **Why it matters.** The Strain-Counterstrain curriculum covers approximately 200 techniques across two primary courses. The Fascial Counterstrain curriculum adds over 900 techniques across six anatomical systems. That's the scale of what you would be taking on, and it's the reason clinicians describe this as a multi-year path rather than a weekend certification.
>
> **What you walk away with.** The eligibility rules, the sequence, and a clear view of the practice-model consequences.

Who can train

A state-issued healthcare license is required. The Jones Institute requires it because the curriculum assumes advanced anatomy and physiology knowledge from day one.

Eligible professions include, and aren't limited to:

↳ Physical therapists and physical therapist assistants

↳ Occupational therapists

↳ Massage therapists

↳ Osteopathic physicians and physicians

↳ Chiropractors

↳ Certified athletic trainers

↳ Other licensed healthcare practitioners

The Jones Institute is an approved continuing education provider with the National Certification Board for Therapeutic Massage and Bodywork, which matters for massage therapists tracking CE credit.

If you're a health or wellness practitioner without a state license, the standing answer is that the licensed-clinician requirement applies. Contact the institute directly about current options rather than relying on anything printed in a book.

The two curricula

Strain-Counterstrain

Developed by Lawrence Jones, DO, and Randall Kusunose, PT, OCS. Roughly 200 techniques across two primary courses:

↳ **SCS Complete Body**

↳ **SCS Cranial**

After those, two paths. A mentorship program to develop clinical application one-on-one, or an examination for board certification in Jones Strain Counterstrain.

This is the foundation. If you want a gentle, no-force manual approach to somatic dysfunction without committing to the full fascial curriculum, this is a complete and defensible place to stop.

Fascial Counterstrain

Developed by Brian Tuckey, PT, OCS, JSCCI. Over 900 techniques across six anatomical systems, plus the FCS Cranial Scan, a proprietary whole-body assessment.

The sequence:

FCS Foundations

↳ Position: Prerequisite, take first

↳ What it opens up: Entry to everything below

FCS Musculoskeletal

↳ Position: Advanced

↳ What it opens up: Muscle, joint, ligament

FCS Lymphatic-Venous

↳ Position: Advanced

↳ What it opens up: Drainage, swelling, venous structures

FCS Arterial

↳ Position: Advanced

↳ What it opens up: Arterial fascia, circulation-linked symptoms

FCS Visceral

↳ Position: Advanced

↳ What it opens up: Organs, post-surgical abdominal and pelvic

FCS Nervous System

↳ Position: Advanced

↳ What it opens up: Peripheral nerve, autonomic, sympathetic

Central Sensitization Series

↳ Position: Newer addition

↳ What it opens up: Centrally mediated pain presentations

All Fascial Counterstrain 3-day immersion courses run through the Jones Institute. Mastery-level courses run through the Counterstrain Academy.

Anatomy Dissection

A Counterstrain-specific approach to gross anatomy, with **no prerequisites**, which makes it an unusually good way to evaluate the whole thing before committing.

↳ A 2-day Pelvic Floor course

↳ A 5-day Multi-System course covering musculoskeletal, central nervous system, viscera, and pelvic floor

↳ Maximum student-to-cadaver ratio of six to one

Clinicians who have done this consistently describe it as the single biggest step change in their palpation, whatever technique they practice.

The mastery path

The **Counterstrain Academy** runs the mastery program. The structure is strict and worth understanding before you plan a year.

↳ Each Academy module is designed to follow the corresponding 3-day Jones Institute immersion course.

↳ **Modules must be taken in order.** Module 1, Intro to Counterstrain and the Cranial Scan, comes first.

↳ At registration for each module, you upload your completion certificate from the matching Jones Institute course.

↳ New students register and obtain approval before signing up.

↳ Mentorships are available for one-on-one development.

3D Counterstrain is the digital reference platform. Access tiers are matched to your completed coursework, so you can purchase access equal to your current training level and no higher.

JSCCI, Jones Strain Counterstrain Certified Instructor, is the teaching credential. A small number of people hold it.

What this does to how you run your practice

This is the part the course catalog won't tell you, and it's the deciding factor for most clinicians.

Sessions get longer. Counterstrain treatment typically runs 60 to 90 minutes of undivided one-on-one attention. That's incompatible with a schedule built on overlapping patients and short units.

Reimbursement gets awkward. Manual therapy codes exist, but standard outpatient reimbursement doesn't fund a 90-minute solo session well. Many practitioners who go deep into this end up cash-pay or hybrid, and that's a business decision as much as a clinical one.

Referral patterns change. Practitioners commonly report that once they can address visceral and nervous system fascia, they start receiving the patients other approaches haven't helped yet, which is rewarding and also means a more complex caseload.

The time investment is real. Multiple 3-day courses, travel, tuition, and then the repetition it takes for palpation to become reliable. One course rarely makes anyone competent in this, and good practitioners say so.

Tuition and schedule. Current tuition rates and availability are on the Jones Institute student portal, and the annual course schedule is published as a downloadable PDF. I'm deliberately not printing prices in a book that will outlive them.

The cheapest way to find out whether it suits you

Clinicians who have gone down this path describe the same sequencing problem: the full curriculum is a multi-year commitment, and the thing that decides whether you'll be good at it is palpation aptitude, which nobody can assess from a course catalog.

Two entry points cost the least to be wrong about. Anatomy Dissection has no prerequisites at all, and clinicians consistently report it upgrades their palpation regardless of what they do next. SCS Complete Body is the foundational course, and most people know inside it whether the subtlety suits them.

Some clinicians take to this immediately. Some find the palpation frustrating and don't get reliable at it. Both are legitimate, and one of them is much cheaper to discover early than late.

↳ What would show you whether the palpation suits you, and what's the least expensive way to find that out?

↳ What would a 90-minute appointment do to your schedule, and to your revenue per hour?

↳ Which of your patients would you most want this for, and what would count as it having helped them?

Your Playbook

Copy this section and send it. It stands on its own, with no context from the rest of the book.

> **1.** Confirm your state license qualifies you to register
> *Owner: You · Time: 10 min*

2. Download the current annual course schedule from jicounterstrain.com

Owner: You · Time: 5 min

3. Check tuition and availability in the student portal

Owner: You · Time: 15 min

4. Compare the Anatomy Dissection and SCS Complete Body entry points, neither of which requires the full curriculum

Owner: You · Time: 20 min

5. Receive or observe a session before deciding anything about enrollment

Owner: You · Time: 1 session

6. Model what a 90-minute appointment does to your schedule and your revenue per hour

Owner: You · Time: 60 min

The 3 rules that make it work.

1. **Whether you're any good at the palpation decides this, and no course catalog can tell you.** That's what the cheap entry points are for.
2. **Feeling it happen to you is different from reading about it.** Most clinicians say that's what decided them, either way.

3. **A 90-minute appointment is a business model change, not just a clinical skill.** The schedule math is part of the decision.

How you'll know it's working in 30 days. You've received one session yourself, and you've got a spreadsheet showing what a 90-minute appointment does to your week.

Which of your patients would you most want to resolve rather than manage, and what have you already tried?

CONCLUSION

The Things You Stopped Doing

Chronic pain doesn't take a life in one piece. It takes it in a long series of small, reasonable-sounding decisions that rarely feel like decisions at the time.

What have you stopped doing, and would you start again if the cause were resolved?

Start Here: The 60-Second Version

The decision this chapter helps you make. What, if anything, you want to do with the next month.

The questions it answers.

↳ What was worth carrying out of this book?

↳ What do I actually know now that I didn't before?

↳ How would I tell whether any of this was working?

↳ What do I want back?

Why it matters. In 2023, about 1 in 4 U.S. adults lived with chronic pain, and about 1 in 12 had pain that often limited life or work. Many of them have been told at some point that management was the plan. This book has laid out one technique with a thin but real evidence base, four self-directed approaches with ran-

> domized trials behind them, and the questions that separate a testable plan from an open-ended one.
>
> **What you walk away with.** A short list of what's known, a short list of what nobody knows yet, and your own answer to the last question in this book.

It rarely feels like a decision

Many people describe it the same way. They stop sitting on the floor, because getting up is the problem. They stop booking the aisle seat, because they already know they'll need to stand. They say they're tired instead of saying they hurt, because they've run out of ways to explain it that don't sound like complaining.

There's a line, and it moves in a few inches at a time. It rarely announces itself. One day it's easy to notice where it is now, and how far out it used to be.

That's what this book has really been about. Not the number on a pain scale.

Five things worth carrying out of here

When relief doesn't last, that's a clue, not a verdict. Something that helps for three days got to something real and stopped short of the cause. That tells you where to look next, and it says nothing about whether you can be helped.

The gap is structural, and it belongs to nobody. Counterstrain is taught after graduation, sold through no sales channel, backed by little research funding, and it takes 60 to 90 minutes per patient. That goes a long way toward explaining why a good physician with a full waiting room hasn't mentioned it. No one had to fail at anything for it to be true.

A no-force technique and a scalpel don't deserve the same level of scrutiny. What each one costs to be wrong about is different, and so is what it costs to find out.

Managing something and resolving it are different goals, and you get to pick which one you're working toward. Most of what gets offered for chronic pain has no finish line in it. Work aimed at the cause does, and that's the whole reason to go looking for one.

There are options even where no practitioner works. Movement, tai chi, mindfulness-based stress reduction, pain reprocessing therapy, and slow-paced breathing all have randomized trials behind them. Several of them are free.

What nobody knows yet

Being straight about this is the whole reason the rest of the book is worth anything.

↳ Whether Fascial Counterstrain outperforms a sham manual technique. No trial has tested it.

↳ How durable the results are in musculoskeletal pain. The longest controlled follow-up is 6 months, in PTSD.

↳ Whether the visceral, vascular, and autonomic applications hold up. Those rest on clinical report.

↳ How much of it is the technique and how much is 90 uninterrupted minutes with someone who took a full history. That question has never been isolated, and it's the most interesting one in the field.

Anyone calling those settled has gone past what's known.

The questions worth asking yourself

I can't know your history, your diagnosis, or what you've already carried, so I've stayed out of the business of telling you what to do next.

What I can do is hand you the questions. They're the more useful half anyway.

↳ What has the last year of managing this actually cost, counting the parts that never showed up on a bill?

↳ What would need to change, and by how much, for it to have been worth finding out?

↳ Who would notice first if something changed?

↳ What would tell you, inside a month, that a direction was wrong?

↳ What would you want to have tried, if you look back on this year from the far side of it?

People often find the last one is the easiest to answer, and the hardest to un-know afterward.

The part that isn't about pain

I don't know your case, and I'm not going to pretend otherwise. Some pain has a cause that no gentle technique will ever touch. Some of it needs a surgeon or a rheumatologist, and this book has tried to say so plainly every time it came up.

What I'll say instead is this.

The reason anybody chases an answer isn't the pain score. It's the grandchild they don't get down on the floor with. It's the hand they don't reach for on a walk, because they're concentrating on a hip. It's the version of them that other people used to get, before so much attention got quietly reassigned to managing something.

That person isn't gone. They're spending most of their energy somewhere else right now, and they deserve some of it back.

Hope is never wasted. It's usually just waiting on a better map.

Your Playbook

Copy this section and send it. It stands on its own, with no context from the rest of the book.

> **1.** Answer the red flag checklist in Chapter 5 and take anything on it to a physician
>
> *Owner: You · Time: 10 min*

> **2.** Write the full injury, surgery, and illness timeline, oldest first
>
> *Owner: You · Time: 25 min*

> **3.** Pick one repeatable movement and record today's number
>
> *Owner: You · Time: 5 min*

> **4.** Write down what would tell you, inside 30 days, that a direction is wrong
>
> *Owner: You · Time: 10 min*

> **5.** Answer the last question in this book, out loud, to somebody
>
> *Owner: You · Time: 5 min*

The 3 rules that make it work.

1. **Red flags outrank everything in this book.** Always, and first.
2. **Write the timeline before anyone asks for it.** You're the only one who has it.
3. **Decide in advance what would change your mind.** That's what keeps this from turning into a standing appointment.

How you'll know it's working in 30 days. One measured movement has a second number next to it, and you can say what that number means.

Who in your life is living with pain they've been told to manage, and what would it mean to pass this on?

Quick Answers

Need one answer without rereading a chapter? These are the questions people ask most, answered in a paragraph each.

What is Fascial Counterstrain?

A gentle, hands-on technique. A trained practitioner finds small tender points linked to deeper tissue, positions the body so that tissue goes slack for about 30 to 90 seconds, then rechecks. There's no force and no cracking. It grew out of Strain-Counterstrain, developed by osteopathic physician Lawrence Jones in the 1950s.

Does it hurt?

It shouldn't. The method depends on tissue letting go when it isn't being fought, so a painful position usually means the position is wrong. Some people feel mild soreness for a day afterward, like after unfamiliar exercise.

How many sessions does it take?

Clinics that provide it commonly describe a handful, often 1 to 6 for a primary complaint. That figure is clinic-reported. The one randomized study used 3 sessions of 90 minutes, and the effect held for 6 months, in PTSD rather than back pain.

Is Counterstrain legit, and is there research behind it?

It's a real, decades-old technique taught to licensed clinicians, and the evidence is mixed. Fascial Counterstrain has one small randomized trial, in PTSD with 22 people analyzed, from authors with a financial stake. Its parent technique has a set of small trials: some favorable, and some, including the largest, in acute low back pain, showing no added benefit. Promising in places, unproven overall, low risk.

Does insurance cover it?

Sometimes. Many practitioners are physical therapists who bill standard manual therapy codes. Others are out of network and provide a superbill. HSA and FSA funds generally cover physical therapy from a licensed provider, and a quick call to the plan confirms it. Medicare Part B covers medically necessary outpatient physical therapy from Medicare-enrolled providers, and some cash-only clinics aren't enrolled, so that's worth asking before booking.

How is it different from massage, chiropractic, or dry needling?

Counterstrain uses no force and aims at tender points linked to deeper tissue, often away from the pain. Massage works muscle near the pain, chiropractic adjusts joints with a quick thrust, dry needling targets trigger points, and physical therapy builds strength and movement. Chapter 3 has them side by side.

Can it help if my MRI is normal?

A normal scan rules out a lot, and that's worth having. It can't see irritation in connective tissue. About 85% of chronic back pain has no clear cause on exam or imaging, which is the zone this model is built for.

How do I find a practitioner?

The Jones Institute directory and the Counterstrain Academy clinic finder list trained clinicians in 41 states plus DC and 8 countries, as of 2026. The most useful question before booking: which courses have you completed, and do you treat the visceral and nervous systems?

Is it normal to feel sore or worse afterward?

Often, and briefly. Across hands-on therapies, mild short-lived reactions follow about 1 in 5 treatments in randomized trials, and serious events are rare. Anything on the Chapter 5 red-flag list, or pain still climbing after about 3 days, is worth a call to a clinician. Chapter 3 has more.

Can I do Counterstrain on myself?

Simple muscle positioning is low risk, and a physician-written self-help version exists, but no trial has tested self-treatment. The deeper visceral and nervous-system work needs a trained practitioner. Chapter 7 covers what helps between sessions.

How is it different from myofascial release or craniosacral therapy?

Myofascial release uses sustained pressure and stretch on tissue near the pain. Craniosacral therapy uses very light touch, mostly on the head, spine, and pelvis. Counterstrain shortens the tissue around a tender point and holds it there, with light glides at most. Chapter 3 has the full comparison.

Which of these would you want someone you care about to know before their next appointment?

Find a Practitioner and Other Resources

Every link is printed in full, so it works whether you're holding paper or a screen.

Counterstrain, main site
counterstrain.com

Find a Counterstrain clinic near you
academy.counterstrain.com/clinics

Jones Institute practitioner directory
jicounterstrain.configio.com/accountdirectory

Counterstrain training for licensed clinicians
jicounterstrain.com/courses

Counterstrain course schedule and tuition
jicounterstrain.com

Find a pain reprocessing therapist
painreprocessingtherapy.com

Free First Visit Kit: timeline template, 5 questions, stop rule
LeadWithGold.com/first-visit-kit

Free articles on chronic pain and more
LeadWithGold.com/blog

The Lead With Gold newsletter

LeadWithGold.com/newsletters/lead-with-gold-newsletter

Free resources, summaries, and the rest of my books

LeadWithGold.com/books

If a link ever stops working, start at counterstrain.com for anything about the technique, and at LeadWithGold.com for anything about this book.

About the Author

Ever been told there's nothing more anyone can do?

Keryn Gold, PhD, MBA has heard some version of that, and so have people she cares about. For 20 years it was her own knee. She'd filed the pain under things you live with, until a friend mentioned a technique she'd never heard of. She read the research first, the way a scientist does, then booked one appointment. The knee pain she'd carried since she was a teenager resolved, and so did longstanding back pain after it.

That's why this book exists. She wanted the next person to have the visibility and access she didn't have for two decades, along with an honest map of what the evidence does and doesn't show.

She finds the outside-the-box solutions most people don't have visibility or access to. She holds a PhD in Biomedical Sciences and Statistical Genetics from Washington University in St. Louis, where she started college at 14 and graduated summa cum laude at 17. She also holds an MBA.

She built the data science and health economics and outcomes research centers of excellence for some of the largest healthcare organizations in the country. She has hired, mentored, and empowered teams at FAANG companies, served as CEO and COO of multiple companies, and worked as a venture capital and private equity operator alongside founders and finance executives.

Across her career, that work has added up to over $3 billion in savings. Those savings weren't from layoffs or cutting quality. They came from improving things for her clients, employees, and patients.

She empowers others through deep diligence and crafts actionable solutions with Day 1 ROI. Creating win-wins everywhere she goes is the throughline.

This is one of a collection of highly rated books from Amazon bestselling author Keryn Gold, on solutions you haven't had visibility or access to previously.

At home, she's outnumbered by her husband, her son, and 2 rescue dogs, one of whom treats a sunny spot on the floor as a full-time job.

What's one thing you'd love to say yes to again?

One additional quick note. To paraphrase one of my favorite fantasy authors:

> *"Reviews are like hugs: Occasionally awkward, but always appreciated."*

If something in here was helpful, an honest review enables the next person who's feeling stuck to find it.

Thanks for reading. I hope this gave you an action plan that empowers you, and I look forward to hearing your story.

To join the newsletter and stay up to date on the latest empowering tools and action plans we have to offer as the market evolves, click here.

For FB silliness, click here: facebook.com/ileadwithgold.

For Instagram ridiculousness, here's a link: instagram.com/leadwithgold.

You can also follow us here:

↳ LinkedIn: linkedin.com/company/lead-with-gold

↳ YouTube: youtube.com/@leadwithgold

↳ TikTok: tiktok.com/@ileadwithgold

↳ X: x.com/LeadwithGold

↳ Threads: threads.com/@leadwithgold

↳ Pinterest: pinterest.com/leadwithgold

↳ Bluesky: bsky.app/profile/leadwithgold.bsky.social

Also by Keryn Gold, PhD, MBA

Empowering you to achieve what you once thought impossible

Tap any title to learn more, or find them all at LeadWithGold.com/books.

From Invisible to Undeniable Get seen. Get understood. Get hired. How to take control of your career path when AI is reading the resumes and writing them too.

The Leadership Playbook, Revisited How to accelerate success, guide and empower your people, navigate change, and build good AI habits to take control of your work life and future-proof your career, today.

From "Misunderstood, Quiet, Introverted, Empathic, Highly Sensitive Person" to "Undeniable, Impactful, Changemaker" How to harness your gifts to do more good and own your future, without losing yourself.

Personalized Learning Made Easy: Empowering Students with AI A how-to guide to set your kids up for success, improve engagement, boost outcomes, and unlock your child's potential with adaptive AI coaching.

Teaching and Education Without Burnout How AI tools empower teachers, future-proof students, enable innovation, unlock personalized learning, save time, improve outcomes, and reignite a love of learning.

The Root Cause of Your Symptoms, Uncovered Why a normal blood test doesn't always rule out a deficiency inside the cell, and what can help with persistent symptoms.

Gut Health Breakthrough What the research says about your microbiome, inflammation, and fatigue, and what you can do with it.

Don't Just Survive, Thrive and Defy Limits Building resilience and capability when the conditions aren't what you would have chosen.

Mind-Blowing Connections For Kids! The Book of Interesting, Weird-But-True Fun Science Facts Why Earth, space, plants, animals, and the brains of smart, curious children share surprising links.

For a free detailed summary of any of these, scan the code or visit LeadWithGold.com/freegift

References and Sources

Grouped by chapter. Where a source has a financial interest in the thing it measures, that is noted here as well as in the text.

Fascial Counterstrain: primary sources

Christy H, Tuckey B, Miljacic N, Polissar N, Vythilingam M. Rapid reduction in posttraumatic stress disorder symptom severity after three fascial counterstrain manual treatments: a proof-of-concept study. Military Medicine. 2026;191(3-4):e513 to e521. Published online 13 August 2025. doi:10.1093/milmed/usaf408
Open access. Two authors own clinics providing the treatment and are paid instructors for the organization that sells the training; the developer of the technique is an author. Funded by the Bridge Back Project, a nonprofit.

Koura GM, Elshiwi AM, Selim M, Asiri AA, Alqahtani RH, Elimy D, Alshehri MA, Alnakhli HH, Assiri SM, Ahmad F, Ahmad I. Comparing the therapeutic impact of strain-counterstrain and exercise on low back myofascial pain syndrome: a randomized trial. Journal of Multidisciplinary Healthcare. 2025;18:1 to 12. doi:10.2147/JMDH.S499927 *n=30. A methodological critique letter was published in the same journal, 2025;18:469 to 471, doi:10.2147/JMDH.S516790.*

Tuckey B, et al. Immediate quantitative sensory testing of the fascial counterstrain method: a case study. Lymphatics. 2026;4(2):17. doi:10.3390/lymphatics4020017

Single case report. The developer of the technique is an author. Ethical approval was waived because a single case report does not meet the definition of human-subjects research.

Kim J. Immediate neuromuscular and functional responses to fascial distortion model and strain-counterstrain in individuals with latent upper trapezius myofascial trigger points: a randomized pilot study. Journal of Manual and Manipulative Therapy. Published online 11 July 2026. doi: 10.1080/10669817.2026.2701346 *n=20 healthy adults. Found no difference between the two techniques. The author declared no conflict of interest and no funding. No untreated control group.*

Bridge Back Project. Research. bridgeback.org/research
The nonprofit that funded the PTSD trial. States that Fascial Counterstrain is not an approved treatment for PTSD and is considered experimental.

Tuckey B, Srbely J, Rigney G, Vythilingam M, Shah J. Impaired lymphatic drainage and interstitial inflammatory stasis in chronic musculoskeletal and idiopathic pain syndromes: exploring a novel mechanism. Frontiers in Pain Research. 2021;2:691740. doi:10.3389/fpain.2021.691740
Theoretical mechanism review, not a clinical trial. The lead author developed Fascial Counterstrain.

Tuckey B. Fascial Counterstrain: a methodological advancement in indirect osteopathic manipulation. International Journal of Osteopathic Medicine. 2025;58:100789. doi: 10.1016/j.ijosm.2025.100789

The author declares ownership of the copyrights on the techniques described.

Tuckey B, Shah JP, Tandon H. A new rationale and treatment model for neuromuscular tender points: case study and developmental history of fascial counterstrain therapy. Self-published white paper, Tuckey Continuing Education Services; 2017. Hosted at counterstrain.com.

Jones LH, Kusunose R, Goering E. Jones Strain-Counterstrain. Boise: Jones Strain Counterstrain Incorporated; 1995.

Strain-Counterstrain and positional release: controlled trials and reviews

Lewis C, Souvlis T, Sterling M. Strain-Counterstrain therapy combined with exercise is not more effective than exercise alone on pain and disability in people with acute low back pain: a randomised trial. Journal of Physiotherapy. 2011;57(2):91 to 98. doi:10.1016/S1836-9553(11)70019-4

Klein R, Bareis A, Schneider A, Linde K. Strain-counterstrain to treat restrictions of the mobility of the cervical spine in patients with neck pain: a sham-controlled randomized trial. Complementary Therapies in Medicine. 2013;21(1):1 to 7. doi:10.1016/j.ctim.2012.11.003

Segura-Ortí E, Prades-Vergara S, Manzaneda-Piña L, Valero-Martínez R, Polo-Traverso JA. Trigger point dry needling versus strain-counterstrain technique for upper trapezius myofascial trigger points: a randomised controlled trial. Acupuncture in Medicine. 2016;34(3):171 to 177. doi: 10.1136/acupmed-2015-010868

Wong CK, Abraham T, Karimi P, Ow-Wing C. Strain counterstrain technique to decrease tender point palpation pain compared to control conditions: a systematic review with meta-analysis. Journal of Bodywork and Movement Therapies. 2014;18(2):165 to 173. doi:10.1016/j.jbmt.2013.09.010

Danazumi MS, Zakari UU, Yakasai AM, Speicher TE, Dermody G, Hassan AB. Positional release technique in the management of low back pain: a systematic review and meta-analysis. Journal of Bodywork and Movement Therapies. 2025;44:295 to 311. doi:10.1016/j.jbmt.2025.05.021
One author is affiliated with the Positional Release Therapy Institute.

El-Khateeb YS, Mahmoud AG, Mohamed MH, Abd El-Azeim AS. Influence of adding strain-counterstrain to standard therapy on axioscapular muscles amplitude and fatigue in mechanical neck pain: a single-blind, randomized trial. European Journal of Physical and Rehabilitation Medicine. 2022;58(4):621 to 629. doi:10.23736/S1973-9087.22.07194-5

Ghanbari A, Rahimijaberi A, Mohamadi M, Abbasi L, Sarvestani FK. The effect of trigger point management by positional release therapy on tension type headache. NeuroRehabilitation. 2012;30(4):333 to 339. doi:10.3233/NRE-2012-0764

Mohamadi M, Rojhani-Shirazi Z, Assadsangabi R, Rahimi-Jaberi A. Can the positional release technique affect central sensitization in patients with chronic tension-type headache? A randomized clinical trial. Archives of Physical Medicine and Rehabilitation. 2020;101(10):1696 to 1703. doi:10.1016/j.apmr.2020.05.028

Wynne MM, Burns JM, Eland DC, Conatser RR, Howell JN. Effect of counterstrain on stretch reflexes, Hoffmann reflexes, and clinical outcomes in subjects with plantar fasciitis. Journal of the American Osteopathic Association. 2006;106(9):547 to 556.

Collins CK, Masaracchio M, Cleland JA. The effectiveness of strain counterstrain in the treatment of patients with chronic ankle instability: a randomized clinical trial. Journal of Manual and Manipulative Therapy. 2014;22(3):119 to 128. doi: 10.1179/2042618614Y.0000000069

Safety and self-care

Carnes D, Mars TS, Mullinger B, Froud R, Underwood M. Adverse events and manual therapy: a systematic review. Manual Therapy. 2010;15(4):355 to 363. doi:10.1016/j.math.2009.12.006

Counterstrain. Occupational stress. counterstrain.com/?p=5568
The technique's own site; source of the note on memories during or after treatment.

Dahm KT, Brurberg KG, Jamtvedt G, Hagen KB. Advice to rest in bed versus advice to stay active for acute low-back pain and sciatica. Cochrane Database of Systematic Reviews. 2010;(6):CD007612. doi:10.1002/14651858.CD007612.pub2

Anderson DL. Muscle Pain Relief in 90 Seconds: The Fold and Hold Method. New York: John Wiley & Sons. ISBN 978-0-471-34689-0.

Self-help book by a physician. Not a research publication; cited as the self-applied adaptation described in Chapter 7.

Fascia and the interstitium

Benias PC, Wells RG, Sackey-Aboagye B, Klumpers D, Wang H, DelGiorno KE, et al. Structure and distribution of an unrecognized interstitium in human tissues. Scientific Reports. 2018;8:4947. doi:10.1038/s41598-018-23062-6

Schleip R, Müller DG. Training principles for fascial connective tissues: scientific foundation and suggested practical applications. Journal of Bodywork and Movement Therapies. 2013;17(4):390 to 398. doi:10.1016/j.jbmt.2013.06.002

Imaging and asymptomatic findings

Brinjikji W, Luetmer PH, Comstock B, Bresnahan BW, Chen LE, Deyo RA, et al. Systematic literature review of imaging features of spinal degeneration in asymptomatic populations. American Journal of Neuroradiology. 2015;36(4):811 to 816. doi:10.3174/ajnr.A4173

Chronic pain prevalence

Lucas JW, Sohi I. Chronic pain and high-impact chronic pain in U.S. adults, 2023. NCHS Data Brief, no. 518. Hyattsville, MD: National Center for Health Statistics; November 2024. doi:10.15620/cdc/169630

Self-directed and mind-body interventions

Wang C, Schmid CH, Fielding RA, Harvey WF, Reid KF, Price LL, Driban JB, Kalish R, Rones R, McAlindon T. Effect of tai chi versus aerobic exercise for fibromyalgia: comparative effectiveness randomized controlled trial. BMJ. 2018;360:k851. doi:10.1136/bmj.k851

Cherkin DC, Sherman KJ, Balderson BH, Cook AJ, Anderson ML, Hawkes RJ, Hansen KE, Turner JA. Effect of mindfulness-based stress reduction vs cognitive behavioral therapy or usual care on back pain and functional limitations in adults with chronic low back pain: a randomized clinical trial. JAMA. 2016;315(12):1240 to 1249. doi:10.1001/jama.2016.2323

Ashar YK, Gordon A, Schubiner H, Uipi C, Knight K, Anderson Z, Carlisle J, Polisky L, Geuter S, Flood TF, Kragel PA, Dimidjian S, Lumley MA, Wager TD. Effect of pain reprocessing therapy vs placebo and usual care for patients with chronic back pain: a randomized clinical trial. JAMA Psychiatry. 2022;79(1):13 to 23. doi:10.1001/jamapsychiatry.2021.2669
Several authors disclose commercial relationships with pain treatment companies. Source of the figure that about 85% of chronic back pain is primary. A critique of the control conditions was published in the same journal, 2022;79(3):271 to 272.

Breathing

Laborde S, Allen MS, Borges U, Dosseville F, Hosang TJ, Iskra M, et al. Effects of voluntary slow breathing on heart rate and heart rate variability: a systematic review and a meta-analysis. Neuroscience and Biobehavioral Reviews. 2022;138:104711. doi:10.1016/j.neubiorev.2022.104711

Nestor J. Breath: The New Science of a Lost Art. Riverhead Books; 2020.
Trade non-fiction, not a research publication. Cited here as the popular source of several claims evaluated in Chapter 9.

Bentley TGK, D'Andrea-Penna G, Rakic M, Arce N, LaFaille M, Berman R, Cooley K, Sprimont P. Breathing practices for stress and anxiety reduction: conceptual framework of implementation guidelines based on a systematic review of the published literature. Brain Sciences. 2023;13(12):1612. doi: 10.3390/brainsci13121612

Remote musculoskeletal care

Peterson Health Technology Institute. Virtual Musculoskeletal Solutions: Health Technology Assessment. June 2024. phti.org/assessment/virtual-msk-solutions
Independent assessment organization. Does not sell any of the evaluated solutions.

Cui D, et al. Randomized controlled trial assessing a digital care program versus conventional physiotherapy for chronic low back pain. npj Digital Medicine. 2023;6:121. doi: 10.1038/s41746-023-00870-3

Sponsored by the company whose program was evaluated; several authors are its employees.

Priebe JA, Kerkemeyer L, Haas KK, Achtert K, Moreno Sanchez LF, Stockert P, et al. Medical app treatment of non-specific low back pain in the 12-month cluster-randomized controlled trial Rise-uP: where clinical superiority meets cost savings. Journal of Pain Research. 2024;17:2239 to 2255. doi:10.2147/JPR.S473250 *n=1,237. Two authors disclose consulting relationships with the app company. The intervention was a digital-first care pathway, not the app alone.*

Pak SS, Janela D, Freitas N, Costa F, Moulder RG, Molinos M, Areias AC, Bento V, Cohen SP, Yanamadala V, Souza R, Correia FD. Comparing digital to conventional physical therapy for chronic shoulder pain: randomized controlled trial. Journal of Medical Internet Research. 2023;25:e49236. doi: 10.2196/49236
Authors are employees of the company whose program was evaluated.

Domingues B, et al. Digital versus in-person physical therapy in adults with musculoskeletal conditions: retrospective matched-cohort analysis of surgery and low-value surgical rates. Journal of Medical Internet Research. 2025;27:e82573. doi:10.2196/82573*Retrospective analysis, not a randomized trial. Funded by the company whose program was evaluated; authors are its employees.*

Counterstrain training

The Jones Institute. Courses and curricula. jicounterstrain.com/courses The Jones Institute. Frequently asked questions, including licensing requirements. jicounterstrain.com/faq Counterstrain Academy. Mastery program structure and prerequisites. counterstrain.com/counterstrain-academy/mastery-program-experience Jones Institute practitioner directory. jicounterstrain.configio.com/account-directory Counterstrain Academy clinic finder. academy.counterstrain.com/clinics

www.ingramcontent.com/pod-product-compliance
Lightning Source LLC
LaVergne TN
LVHW010731061126
851857LV00014B/1428
* 9 7 8 1 9 6 7 4 5 6 1 9 2 *